"A wise and compassionate book that illuminates how trauma survivors can finally make peace with emotional eating. Diane Petrella guides readers to deeply understand why their trauma has led to their struggles—and offers healing strategies, wisdom, and gentle kindness to release their pain, secrets, anxiety, and stress. Petrella captures the heartbeat of what it means to recover from trauma and emotional eating, and offers hope that recovery is possible."

—**Mary Anne Cohen, LCSW, BCD**, director of The New York Center for Eating Disorders; and author of three books on eating disorders, including *Lasagna for Lunch*

"I wish I had this book thirty-five years ago when I started on my own journey toward making peace with food and my body. If you're ready to develop a more compassionate understanding of how your emotional eating helps you cope with developmental trauma, and experience a nourishing relationship with food, Diane is your guide! *Healing Emotional Eating for Trauma Survivors* is clear and comprehensive, filled with heart and inspiration."

—**Barbara L. Holtzman, MSW, LICSW**, psychotherapist; and author of *Conscious Eating, Conscious Living*

"*Healing Emotional Eating for Trauma Survivors* is a gentle tour de force of a book. From its first words, seasoned therapist Diane Petrella guides readers onto a path of compassionate self-healing of the trauma that lies within emotional eating. Her knowledge base is deep and wide, and her therapeutic approaches address mind, body, and soul, opening doors for all to make new choices."

—**Joanne Ahola, MD, DLFAPA**, psychiatrist in New York City, NY; specializing in psychotherapy and the psychological effects of trauma and human rights abuses

T0026593

"This deeply compassionate look at the connection between early trauma and emotional eating provides an outstanding self-help program for addressing these painful issues. With warmth and empathy, Diane Petrella guides you along a path of healing that is based on empirical data and clinical wisdom. As you travel this journey, you'll feel as if Diane is holding your hand, offering reassurance and comfort every step of the way."

—**Leigh Anne Hohlstein, PhD**, clinical assistant professor in
the department of psychiatry and human behavior at the
Warren Alpert Medical School at Brown University, and
psychotherapist specializing in the treatment of eating disorders

"*Healing Emotional Eating for Trauma Survivors* offers practical and grounded strategies to help you heal 'both inside-out and outside-in.' If you are a trauma survivor—this kind and gentle book will help you have a greater understanding of the impact of your trauma on your emotional system, and have a better relationship with your body and food."

—**Gretchen L. Schmelzer, PhD**, author of *Journey
Through Trauma*

"Diane Petrella brings a compassionate approach to resolving the challenges of emotional eating and childhood trauma. She provides many nourishing practices to establish a healthy relationship with food, while gently addressing early trauma. Diane's step-by-step guidance, prompts, and suggestions can bring you back to a deep sense of security, opening you to your innermost being."

—**Julie Brown Yau, PhD**, author of *The Body Awareness
Workbook for Trauma*

"If you're a trauma survivor and use food to cope, you'll find comfort, guidance, and hope in this insightful book. Petrella helps you understand that emotional eating *is not your fault*, but a self-care strategy that helped you survive. She then compassionately guides you through easy, comforting strategies you can use to heal emotionally, rebalance your nervous system, and discover your authentic self as you find freedom from emotional eating."

—**Courtney Armstrong, LPC**, author of *Rethinking Trauma Treatment*

"Practical, smart, and wise, this beautifully crafted guide fills a much-neglected niche in the trauma self-help literature. Diane succeeds in de-pathologizing and simplifying the complexities of emotional, cognitive, somatic, and behavioral residue of trauma. She offers simple yet powerful practices for addressing the nervous system dysregulation that leads to emotional eating. Readers will discover new ways of dealing with triggering states, resulting in more resilience and adaptive behaviors. Highly recommended!"

—**Julie M. Simon, MA, MBA, LMFT**, licensed psychotherapist, life coach, and author of *The Emotional Eater's Repair Manual* and *When Food Is Comfort*

"Diane Petrella's compassionate voice comes through loud and clear in this excellent book that examines the connection between emotional eating and trauma. With an understanding that turning to food for comfort isn't about a lack of willpower, a matter of addiction, or solved through dieting, Diane offers practical, gentle strategies to heal your relationship with food at any size."

—**Judith Matz, LCSW**, coauthor of *The Diet Survivor's Handbook* and *The Making Peace with Food Card Deck*

Healing Emotional Eating
for Trauma Survivors

**Trauma-Informed Practices to
Nurture a Peaceful Relationship with
Your Emotions, Body, and Food**

Diane Petrella, MSW

New Harbinger Publications, Inc.

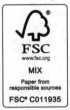

Copyright © 2023 by Diane Petrella
New Harbinger Publications, Inc.
5674 Shattuck Avenue
Oakland, CA 94609
www.newharbinger.com

The music used in the downloadable audio meditations is "The River of Love" by Thaddeus from OrinDaben.com. Used with permission.

Cover design by Amy Shoup

Acquired by Georgia Kolias

Edited by Gretel Hakanson

Library of Congress Cataloging-in-Publication Data on file

Printed in the United States of America

25   24   23

10   9   8   7   6   5   4   3   2   1   First Printing

To my clients, who welcomed me into their hearts.
This book is for you, with love.

Contents

Foreword

Healing Emotional Eating for Trauma Survivors is a breakthrough tool to help you make the crucial, life-changing connection between emotional eating and early trauma. In this sensitive, passionate guide to healing emotional eating, Diane takes you on a personal, handheld journey. And a timely one. Today, more than ever, the messages girls and women receive—especially online—are body-centric, focusing on narrow parameters for female beauty and appearance. It's not surprising that women are likely to turn these external societal messages against themselves and internalize them in ways that can show up as self-criticism, self-loathing, and disordered eating. Men, too, receive messages about what constitutes acceptable masculinity and the ideal male body, which can leave them feeling inadequate. Our society's body-centric messaging affects all individuals wherever they are on the gender spectrum.

But this is especially the case in people with a history of trauma.

When children and teens experience trauma or adversity without adequate adult support, and that trauma is kept secret or isn't openly addressed, children code this to mean that there must be something wrong with *them*. If you experience childhood adversity and the adults in your life don't have your back or help you understand what is happening, you can live a lifetime feeling that what happened to you must have been your fault.

As an adult, this can emerge as a deep interior belief that *you* are wrong. Your body is wrong. What you say and do and think is wrong. You may feel full of shame and self-blame because the experiences you endured early in life sent you that message as a child or teen—when you were too young to question it—and that message has not yet been examined and rewritten.

This book helps you make that essential leap to understand that there is nothing wrong with you. There is nothing wrong with who you are.

Most books on emotional eating focus on food, eating mindfully, and intuitive eating without addressing underlying trauma. Diane helps you understand that emotional eating is not about food. It's not your fault if you're having a hard time healing emotional eating. This isn't about your lack of willpower.

We are shaped in countless ways by our early experiences. Traumatic experiences change the architecture of the brain and nervous system in ways that, over time, have a profound effect on our self-beliefs and feelings. These inner beliefs about ourselves, in turn, influence our behaviors. When your nervous system has been primed since childhood to be on high alert because of events in the past, the parts of the brain that help regulate the stress response and allow for clear thinking and decision-making can go offline when you meet up with stress in adult life. It can feel as if your mind has been hijacked, clouding your judgment. And this can affect your relationship with food.

Diane offers you powerful steps and strategies to help you understand why you may be vulnerable to emotional eating, why you may have a hard time changing this pattern even when you try, and why it all comes down to this: you can't truly heal emotional eating without addressing your early trauma. You can't be who you hope to become without taking this journey into yourself and your past so that you can redefine your future.

Diane approaches this sensitive topic from the authoritative, clinical perspective of a licensed psychotherapist, with all the skills and wisdom to help you go at your own pace and succeed every step of the way.

By making this connection and using the neuroscience and evidence-based psychotherapeutic strategies you'll learn in these pages, you will begin to free yourself from the ways trauma has held you hostage and affected your relationship with food. In the process, you will connect with what Diane calls your inner Wise Self for guidance and tap into new spiritual insights, helping you create change from the "inside-out." Ultimately, this is the path to deep and lasting healing.

You're about to embark on a powerful, self-healing journey, one which will afford you a new understanding of not only the wisdom you hold within but also help you rewrite the story of who you really are. The child you once were—your inner child, who so deeply wanted and needed comfort and understanding—will find long-overdue comfort in these pages, and experience, at last, the freedom to release guilt and shame.

With Diane by your side, you are in warm and compassionate hands, and you are never alone.

Here's to your healing journey.

—Donna Jackson Nakazawa
   Author of *Girls on the Brink*, *The Angel and the Assassin*,
   and *Childhood Disrupted*, and creator of the online narrative
   writing program Breaking Free From Trauma

Welcome

I'm so glad you're here.

If you use food as your main way to cope with stress and painful feelings and you endured emotional, physical, or sexual abuse, neglect, or other early trauma, you're in the right place.

And you're not alone.

The emotional and physiological effects of childhood trauma are difficult to deal with, so it makes sense that you look for ways to cope. Despite what you may think, turning to food is *not* a lack of willpower. You've probably tried many times and ways to stop. But if you haven't yet learned about the effects of trauma on your mind, body, and spirit, it's understandable that ending emotional eating has been fraught with struggle.

This book will help. I welcome you to join me on a healing journey that explores the connection between early trauma and emotional eating and offers practices to help you heal.

Research shows that women who experienced childhood physical and sexual abuse were almost *twice as likely* to have a food addiction in adulthood compared to those who were not abused as children (Mason et al. 2013). The Adverse Childhood Experiences Study (ACES), conducted in the mid-1990s by Kaiser Permanente and the Centers for Disease Control and Prevention (CDC), and led by Vincent Felitti, MD and Robert Anda, MD, explored the connection between traumatic childhood experiences and later physical and mental health issues. The results of this large public-health study reveal a direct link between childhood trauma and later chronic illness; addictive behaviors, including food addiction; and other mental health issues. Based on these and other studies, coupled with my clinical experience, it seems futile to address emotional eating without addressing the effects of trauma. That's why I wrote this book for you.

Let me tell you about myself. Early in my nearly forty-year career as a clinical social worker and licensed psychotherapist, I codeveloped the first child sexual-abuse treatment program in Rhode Island. I worked with child and adolescent victims, adults molested as children, and sexual offenders, and conducted expert-witness forensic evaluations on sexual assault and post-traumatic stress disorder cases. My clinical work expanded to all forms of early abuse, neglect, and other adverse childhood experiences, including death, divorce, and having a family member with a mental illness or substance abuse problem. It was during this time that I noticed the connection between early trauma and emotional eating. I worked with many people, mostly women, who used food to cope with pain too hard to bear. It wasn't *really* about the food. It was about the pain—the pain of negative self-worth that lived in my traumatized clients' minds, the sadness held in their heavy hearts, and the unsettling, fear-based sensations of trauma trapped within their bodies. Mostly, they didn't feel safe.

While I work only with adults now, our relationship includes their inner child too. That's the part of them—and I imagine the part of you too—that still feels vulnerable, unprotected, and easily triggered. And I address how my clients feel in their bodies, because unprocessed traumatic pain lives in the nervous system. Think of your body as the container for your emotions. Unprocessed trauma-based emotions can result in what's called body dysregulation, which means you feel unsettling physical sensations ranging from anxiety and fear to disconnection and detachment. Dysregulation is a common physiological effect of early trauma and one reason why you may easily feel triggered to eat. It's important to address the impact of trauma and fear on your body to help you truly heal from both trauma and emotional eating.

So why do you and others turn to food? Below are some reasons. As you read this list, notice what applies to you:

"Sometimes life feels too hard. Eating helps me cope."

"When I'm in a food coma, I don't have to deal with anything."

"When I feel stressed, eating calms me."

"When I feel empty, eating fills the hole in my heart."

"When I feel lonely, food soothes me. It's like I'm with friends."

"I eat to distract myself. Sometimes I just need to check out."

"I eat when I'm angry. But then I get angry at myself for eating."

"I eat to numb my feelings about _____ (my divorce, my husband's death, the argument with my friend, pressure at work, feeling criticized)."

"I eat when I have nothing to do and feel bored."

"I don't even know why. Sometimes I just start eating."

Can you relate to these?

And what happens *after* you eat? Many of my clients end up berating themselves. They beat themselves up with self-criticism and self-loathing. And they feel demoralized, thinking they'll never stop using food to cope.

The thing is, berating yourself after emotionally eating stops you from addressing what triggered you to eat in the first place. You're then unintentionally avoiding dealing with the problem at hand, which can get in the way of deeper healing. For example, many childhood trauma survivors have a hard time prioritizing their self-care. If you feel triggered to eat because you feel resentful about agreeing to babysit your neighbor's child when you already feel overwhelmed, berating yourself for eating shifts your attention away from learning how to set boundaries on your time.

When you try to solve an emotional problem with food, food and eating then become your focus and obscure the deeper emotional issues that need your attention. This book is designed to help you do both: address your impulse to use food when overwhelmed and discover and heal the deeper trauma-related reasons you feel triggered. Because it's not really about food. It's about learning to calm your body's dysregulation and mindfully attending to your feelings and needs so you can truly heal.

So why does food seem to help? Research is inconclusive as to why. Some people may lose their appetite when under emotional stress, and others find that food calms and soothes them. It offers comfort, distraction, and a way to ease hard feelings.

Using food for emotional regulation is defined in different ways. "Emotional eating" is one term, along with "food addiction," "compulsive eating," "binge eating," and "overeating." While there are some differences when it comes to clinical matters in a medical setting, for simplicity's sake, I'll mostly refer to "emotional eating," although I'll sometimes use these other terms too.

Semantics aside, when food has been your main source of comfort, it can feel challenging to stop using food to cope. That's because you're not eating to assuage biological hunger. You're eating to numb the pain in your heart and calm the stress in your body.

Honor yourself for doing the best you can to feel grounded and safe. It's hard to feel deep pain that you fear will never stop. You learned that reaching for food helps you feel better. And it *does* help you feel better, especially when a sugar high or food coma stops you from feeling anything at all—or at least, takes the edge off.

The thing is—and I know you know this—emotional eating is a temporary fix. It doesn't help you feel better for the long term. The feelings you push away still lurk beneath the surface, ready to erupt when you feel stressed at work, frustrated with your partner, sad, lonely—or demoralized because you can't stop emotionally eating—and the cycle continues. And it's not only about your feelings. As mentioned above, trauma affects your body too, so even minor annoyances can trigger unsettling physiological sensations, sometimes without you being consciously aware of it. You then use food to calm your body and don't understand why you felt the impulse to grab that candy bar.

When food is your primary coping tool, three things happen: you get momentary relief while you disconnect yourself from feelings or problems that need your mindful attention, you may eat more than your body needs for its comfort, and you don't effectively address the underlying trauma-related reasons that may have triggered the urge to eat in the first place. You then never get to the deeper issues that allow for sustained healing to happen.

It may feel discouraging to learn about the longstanding effects of childhood trauma, I know. Perhaps you're feeling discouraged just reading this. If so, that's understandable. But knowledge is power. And self-knowledge is freedom. The information in this book offers you an explanation as to why you've struggled with emotional eating for so long. Without this knowledge, you may keep struggling and blame yourself. But with this knowledge, you can find the right solutions. So take heart. Having a history of childhood trauma doesn't mean you can't heal. You *can* heal. And it doesn't mean you can't make peace with food and overcome emotional eating. You can. This book shows you how.

How This Book Will Help You

Many of my clients, and perhaps you too, started turning to food as children or adolescents to cope with the trauma they were enduring. But not all of them started young. Whether you began emotionally eating early in life or later, the underlying reasons are the same, and this book will help.

People of all shapes and sizes emotionally eat. Not everyone who eats for emotional reasons has weight concerns, nor does emotional eating always lead to weight increases. At the same time, some people who struggle with emotional eating also experience body insecurity about their weight. It's possible that some people may release weight once they stop turning to food as their primary way of coping. But weight loss is neither the intention nor promise of this book. The intention is to help you develop a healthier relationship with your feelings, body, and food after struggling with the effects of trauma and emotional eating for so long.

I will address child and adolescent trauma; adverse experiences; and the emotional, developmental, and physiological consequences of them. (For simplicity's sake, however, I may refer to children, but I'm including adolescents too.) If you experienced trauma as an adult and not in childhood and use food to cope, you'll find that the information and practices will be helpful to you too.

This book is for people of any gender but many of my client stories are from the perspective of women as this is the primary makeup of my practice. Women also *appear* to be the main demographic struggling with emotional eating, but I have worked with men too and know that they also struggle with this. They're simply less likely to seek out support the way women do.

Emotional eating and childhood trauma aren't issues you read about and then automatically fix. But going through this process, and putting into practice the exercises you'll be learning, will help move you on the path toward lasting change. This book will not only help you heal emotional eating and early trauma, it also will help you develop compassion for yourself. Because it's not just about what you "do" and the steps you take; it's about *who you become in the process.* And when you become a more self-compassionate person, healing happens.

Support for the Journey Ahead

Chapters 1 and 2 offer you foundational information about early trauma and emotional eating. We'll then address specific themes in chapters 3 through 9: you'll learn how to calm the dysregulation in your nervous system, befriend your body, identify and heal limiting beliefs, mindfully process your feelings, make peace with trigger foods, turn self-punishment into self-compassion, and transform your home into an emotionally safe sanctuary.

I've created a structure for you that progresses from one chapter to the next, so I recommend you read straight through. But everyone learns differently, so if you prefer to read different chapters first, that's fine. Let yourself be drawn to whatever sections resonate with you. You can always repeat steps as needed.

Some of what you read may feel triggering. As you read about others' experiences, you may remember your own. But feeling triggered isn't a reason to avoid something. When you feel triggered, you're offered the promise of growth as you practice new ways to cope and heal. Make the experience of reading cozy and comfortable. Perhaps you'd like to sip a cup of soothing tea or light a candle. Pace yourself and take breaks when needed. I'll be offering you self-calming and grounding tools and asking you to check in with yourself, so feel reassured that I'll be guiding you along the way, along with your Wise Self.

Who is your Wise Self? The invisible, spiritual part of you that is wise, loving, and always guiding you to your highest and best good. Some people describe this part of themselves as their intuition, Spirit, God, or Universe. I'll be using the term "Wise Self" and will suggest that you connect with this part of yourself at different points throughout the book. It's hard to notice your Wise Self's guidance, however, when trauma-based fears live in your mind and body. Nevertheless, trust that your inner Wise Self knew you were ready for another level of healing or you wouldn't have been drawn to this book in the first place. If you have never consciously connected with your Wise Self or want a new way of accessing that part of you, you can download a guided visualization I made for you to meet your Wise Self at the website for this book: http://www.newharbinger.com/51178.

I also made you a relaxation audio. The "Peaceful Place" guided imagery exercise helps you use the power of your mind to create a sanctuary of inner peace. You can use this when you need to pause and take a self-nurture break. Download the audio and read the instruction guide before using the recordings here: http://www.newharbinger.com/51178.

In some of the exercises, I suggest that you close your eyes. For many trauma survivors, however, closing their eyes is triggering because they feel too vulnerable. Staying alert and hypervigilant helps them feel safe. If you feel this way, simply keep your eyes open with a soft downward gaze. Talk with your health care or mental health care provider before starting any practice that may exacerbate a medical or psychiatric challenge that you're facing.

Keep a journal handy to write down your thoughts and feelings as you read. Journal writing is therapeutic and healing. I'm partial to writing by hand because I believe it keeps you more closely connected with your heart energy, but if you prefer using a device, that's okay. Any form of journal writing is powerful.

Healing emotional eating and early trauma is hard to do by yourself. People make smoother progress when they're being supported and witnessed. If you're currently in psychotherapy, you may want to share the practice exercises with your therapist to have their support and guidance. If you've been in therapy in the past, reading this may bring the work you've already done to an even deeper level. If old issues emerge, that's understandable. You may want to consider recontacting your therapist or find someone new to support this phase of your healing. If you've never sought psychotherapy for emotional eating or childhood trauma, perhaps you'll consider working with a licensed psychotherapist to address these issues. (There are tools to find a therapist in the "Resources" section at the back of this book.)

A Support to Use Right Now

Learning to calm your body when dysregulated is a foundational skill for healing both emotional eating and childhood trauma. The good news is that you already possess this ability.

And it's only a breath away.

Diaphragmatic breathing, also called abdominal or belly breathing, is a powerful and simple self-calming technique. The diaphragm is a dome-shaped muscle that sits below your lungs. When fully engaged, it helps pull air into your lungs, increasing blood oxygenation. Diaphragmatic breathing elicits your body's natural relaxation response to help calm your nervous system.

Many people breathe from the upper part of their chest and take short, shallow breaths. I wonder if you do too. Shallow breathing keeps you from getting the full calming effects of each breath, as nature intended.

To discover how you breathe, try this: Sit or stand upright. Place your right hand on your chest and your left hand on your abdomen. Inhale and exhale naturally through your nose and notice which hand is moving more. If the right hand is moving more than the left hand, you're breathing more from your chest. If the left hand is moving more, you're breathing from your diaphragm.

If you breathe from your upper chest, you can train yourself to breathe diaphragmatically.

Once again, sit upright with one hand on your chest and the other on your abdomen. Breathe through your nose. Focus on breathing from deep within your belly. Much like a bellows, which draws air in as it expands and expels air as it contracts, concentrate on expanding your diaphragm as you inhale and contracting it as you exhale. As you do this, you'll notice the hand on your abdomen rising more than the hand on your chest. This is diaphragmatic breathing.

Breathing like this may feel unnatural at first. You, like many people, have probably spent most of your life taking shallow breaths. Shallow breathing is one effect of a hyperalert nervous system. When you're triggered, you can use diaphragmatic breathing—anytime, anywhere—to reregulate and calm your body.

Don't wait to use diaphragmatic breathing only when you're stressed. It's important to practice when you already feel settled. This helps you remember what to do when feeling overwhelmed.

The beauty of diaphragmatic breathing is that it's a handy self-calming tool that's always with you. And no one has to know you're using it. Do your best to breathe when you first notice you're feeling stressed. You can use the following simple five-point body-awareness scale to gauge how calm or unsettled you and your body feel. (You can download a PDF of this scale at http://www.newharbinger.com/51178.)

What number represents how you feel right now?

1 – I feel calm and peaceful.

2 – I feel at ease.

3 – I feel a little unsettled.

4 – I feel very unsettled.

5 – I feel overwhelmed.

When you're at a three on this scale, take five deep and gentle diaphragmatic breaths. This helps you feel calmer and reduces the likelihood that your body becomes highly dysregulated. A calm body helps you feel safe. And when you feel safe, you're more open to learning and using practices to help you heal. To learn how your nervous system communicates calm and stress to you, review this scale several times throughout the day. Use diaphragmatic breathing when necessary.

Early trauma and emotional eating are challenging issues to deal with. Congratulate yourself for having the courage to face them. I know it's not easy. Everyone has a story to tell, and you have yours. While it doesn't have to define you, your story shaped you. Honor that story while creating your next chapter.

I'm honored to walk this journey with you. So let's continue.

CHAPTER 1

Using Food as Self-Protection After Childhood Trauma

Food is nurturance. Along with hugs, gentle words, and the love from a parent's adoring gaze, food and being fed set the early foundation for babies to feel safe and protected knowing that their needs will be met. Receiving food with tender care, from the bottle or breast, becomes a child's first experience of their outer world.

Babies and children are like emotional sponges soaking in the energy around them. In this way their outer world informs their inner world. Trusting that their needs will be met helps babies and children develop inner trust. Experiencing love from caretakers helps them develop self-love. Receiving comfort when distressed helps them experience relief and safety. These nurturing experiences add essential currency into the child's self-worth bank. As children mature, their experiences expand. While their need for food and a safe home life is essential, their self-worth and self-love keep evolving from various sources, such as extended family members, friends, school experiences, social activities, and religious or spiritual traditions. But at its most basic level, the experience of love begins with food.

Food often triggers nostalgic memories. In this way, it *is* emotional. Aunt Betty's holiday apple pie, your grandmother's favorite recipes, or the pizzas your father made for Friday night dinners may elicit warm feelings. That's because food enhances celebrations and family gatherings. These gatherings may be joyous, like a birthday, wedding, or holiday, or mournful as for a funeral. Sometimes parents give their child a special food treat when their child feels distressed. For example, if her child is feeling sad after being rejected by friends, a mother may offer a bowl of ice cream, sit with her child at the kitchen table, and talk about what happened. Using food this way does not start a pattern of emotional eating. When food is woven with a parent's loving attention, the child absorbs the love. Food is extra and pairs with the love already there. But without emotional support, food can become a replacement for love or connection that is absent. Using the above example, if the child lacked support for her painful feelings, food may become her only source of comfort in a lonely, and perhaps unsafe, home.

Take a moment to reflect on your history with food. What are your earliest memories of food and being fed? Do they bring a smile to your face or trigger discomfort? What were mealtimes like growing up? Were they pleasant or fraught with conflict? When did you first start using food to cope with hard feelings? Were you a child or teenager? Or did you not start until you were an adult? If you wish, write about these memories in your journal. And remember to breathe diaphragmatically to settle your nervous system if reflecting on these experiences is painful and triggering.

Food as Comfort

When a child feels sad, anxious, or unsafe and comforting responses from caregivers are absent, they may turn to food for their emotional survival. Unless food is scarce in a child's home, it's often easy to access, candy and chips don't cost too much, and unlike cigarettes or a six-pack of beer, they don't need an ID to purchase it.

When humans hurt, they need relief. If you turned to food for comfort in your early years too, commend yourself because it actually was a resourceful thing to do.

Perhaps your emotional eating challenges did not begin during childhood or adolescence but started later in life. For example, Gail didn't start emotionally eating until her late thirties. That's when she started recovery to stop drinking alcohol. Daily glasses of wine had kept her painful trauma-based feelings at bay. Once she became sober, food replaced her Chardonnay.

If you developed issues with emotional eating later in life, did you previously rely on other substances or behaviors—alcohol, drugs, cigarettes, gambling, sex—to cope? If so, this isn't unusual for survivors of trauma. Until you heal the root cause of your pain, it's hard to free yourself from the ways some substances and behaviors numb that pain.

When I first met Carol, she struggled with emotional eating too. Referred by her dietitian, she tried for years to end this struggle but made little progress. Carol's dietitian had introduced her to the concept of intuitive eating. Carol felt inspired by the idea that she could learn to notice and heed her body's signals to make healthy choices, heal her love-hate relationship with food, and get off the diet roller coaster. She desperately wanted to end obsessing about her weight and worrying about what and when to eat—and when to stop. But as she tried to practice these skills, she just couldn't make it work. She said, "How can I notice my body's needs when I'm filled with anxiety and want to crawl out of my skin?"

Carol's history revealed a traumatic childhood of physical abuse by her mother and sexual abuse by her brother. She learned that hiding sweets and eating them in her bedroom—usually candy bars and cupcakes—relieved her loneliness and fear. Food became Carol's trusted friend, a love-hate relationship that continued into adulthood.

During our work together, Carol learned how her trauma-filled body reacted to stress and how this made her susceptible to emotional eating. She was relieved to learn that this wasn't her fault and she didn't lack willpower. It was because her body was still holding the trauma she endured long ago and easily became triggered today. It didn't take much for Carol's heart to race, muscles to tense, and breathing to quicken. Low-level anxiety was constant and intensified even with minor stress. What Carol had thought was self-sabotage—using food when stressed—was actually rooted in self-protection. Turning to food felt grounding. It took time, but as Carol learned how to calm her body and process her feelings, healing emotional eating became possible. She not only stopped relying on food to cope, but she also began to heal from childhood trauma because these issues were linked.

When food is your emotional life preserver, it's hard to let it go. For example, no matter how much Carol tried to stop eating sweets when she felt lonely and anxious, she just couldn't do it. Cupcakes—Carol's childhood friends—calmed her anxious body, soothed her feelings, and offered a sense of companionship that eased her loneliness. This kind of relationship with food may be hard for some people to understand if they weren't abused and traumatized as children. But it's not unusual at all when your childhood lacked safety and protection and food helped you get through the day. Even if Carol's experience isn't the same as yours, I bet you can relate to how emotionally overwhelmed she felt and why she used food to cope.

So, let's look deeper at where this emotional overwhelm comes from with a mini crash course on brain science and trauma.

How Early Trauma Affects the Brain

Early trauma and abuse create changes in a child and adolescent's developing brain. All early experiences influence brain development. But when a child or teenager suffers chronic trauma and fear, especially within their family, the brain's normal reaction to threats—the fight-flight-freeze response activated by the part of the brain called the amygdala—intensifies. (There's a fourth stress response called fawn that we'll address in chapter 3.)

An overactive amygdala makes you hypersensitive to stress. When triggered, your body and emotions become dysregulated: you feel destabilized, overwhelmed, and experience unsettling sensations in your body. Some of these sensations feel intense; others feel subtle. For example, your heart races; you take rapid breaths; you get a knot in your stomach. You may feel anxious and afraid. Or you feel detached and numb.

Due to early trauma, your brain has been conditioned to be alert for danger, so even low-level stress can activate the fight-flight-freeze response and overwhelm your nervous system. In this dysregulated state, you just want relief—fast. And you've learned that food helps. It's quick, readily available, and eases the overwhelm. When you're in this survival mode, impulse overrides thoughtful reflection. Think about it. If you feel in danger, you don't take time to map out the shortest route to safety—you just run.

And sometimes you run to food.

Learning about your body's response to emotional triggers (which we'll discuss more in chapter 3) will help you heal both emotional eating and early trauma. Noticing these inner sensations and signals is called *interoceptive awareness*, which means knowing the ways your body communicates to you. For example, being aware of how fast or slow you're breathing, whether your muscles feel relaxed or tense, or whether you're hungry or full. Becoming attuned to your body helps you be mindful of what and how much food your body needs. This attunement also helps you recognize your body's signs of stress so you can help it calm down. (Use the body awareness scale that you learned in the "Welcome" section to help you with this.)

The thing is, developing interoceptive awareness may feel hard to master at first when you've experienced early trauma and abuse. That's because the physiological and emotional effects of trauma—unsettling sensations, underlying anxiety, fear, suppressed and repressed memories— stay stored in the body. It can feel overwhelming to notice and tolerate these trauma-based sensations. Simply not having something "to do" may trigger feelings of vulnerability and overwhelm. As Carol said, "*When it gets quiet on the outside, it gets real noisy on the inside.*" Can you relate to that experience?

Bessel van der Kolk (2014, 96–97), world-renowned trauma expert and author of *The Body Keeps the Score: Brain, Mind, and Body in the Healing of Trauma*, describes how trauma lives on in the body:

> *Traumatized people chronically feel unsafe inside their bodies: The past is alive in the form of gnawing interior discomfort. Their bodies are constantly bombarded by visceral warning signs, and in an attempt to control these processes, they often become expert at ignoring their gut feelings and in numbing awareness of what is played out inside. They learn to hide from their selves.*

If you've tried to stop emotionally eating but have been unsuccessful, Dr. van der Kolk's description of the traumatized body explains a major reason why. Noticing and interpreting interoceptive awareness—what's happening in your body—can feel overwhelming and scary, confuse your hunger and fullness signals, and trigger emotional eating.

For example, you've probably noticed that your sensations of physical hunger and emotional hunger sometimes feel intertwined. It's hard to know if you're hungry for dinner when emotional hunger and stress leave you craving for something—*anything*—to fill a deeper void or calm the panic in your body. Grabbing a fast-food burger on your way home from work—after you ate a late lunch—may seem to satisfy your hunger. Or maybe it's numbing the anger triggered by your boss's criticism.

Am I hungry? Or am I angry and scared?

Sometimes it's hard to tell the difference.

For some trauma survivors, turning to food helps protect them from painful memories or flashbacks. Eating comfort foods can distract the mind and block trauma-based memories from surfacing. For example, Grace often was plagued with terrifying memories of her parents' violent fights when she was young. Eating to the point of entering a "food coma" helped block out those frightening pictures invading her mind. Perhaps you've experienced traumatic memories as emotional eating triggers too. It's also possible that you're not consciously aware when this is happening and grabbing something to eat may be an automatic habit your mind uses to keep you emotionally safe. Either way, when you feel destabilized and *don't* turn to food, it's possible that frightening memories may emerge. It's okay to use food when you don't see any other way to feel safe. Food has been your sanctuary for a reason. When you do turn to food, just do your best to eat consciously. For example, you could say, "I'm eating because I feel scared, and nothing else is helping right now." Making eating a *conscious choice* paradoxically helps reduce its power.

So can you heal emotional eating if you have a history of trauma? Of course you can. And learning to feel safe in your body by calming and grounding yourself when stressed will help you make mindful—rather than impulsive—choices. Calming your body activates the relaxation response. And it's the relaxation response that helps you access your intuition so you can make thoughtful choices. Think of it this way:

Your stress response brings you into survival mode. When you're in survival mode, you tend to respond impulsively to triggers. Impulsivity leads to emotional eating.

Your relaxation response—when your body feels calm and settled—allows you to access reflective thinking. You feel safe enough to make mindful—rather than impulsive—choices.

When your body is relaxed, you're not fighting anything. You feel at ease. Your body can communicate its needs, and you're more receptive to that information. That's why using diaphragmatic breathing, which you learned earlier, will help.

Now, relaxing the body can feel hard for trauma survivors. When you're relaxed, you're less vigilant about your surroundings, and this can trigger vulnerability and fear. But this doesn't mean you can't learn to calm your body *and* feel grounded at the same time. You can. It's mostly about *feeling safe* in your body. Later in this chapter, you'll learn another grounding process to add to your self-calming toolbox.

It takes time to heal emotional eating and learn the skills necessary to settle your body, soothe and ground yourself, and let yourself *feel your feelings*. So have patience. I know it may seem hard or scary to do this. It was scary for Carol at first too. When you're triggered with strong emotion (as

Carol was—a lot), it can feel like you're swallowed up with sadness, ready to jump out of your skin with fear, or that your body's on fire with anxiety. Coping with painful feelings is hard—if not impossible—to do when the physiological effects of trauma get triggered in your body. As Carol experienced, she had to first learn how to calm her nervous system before she could tolerate "being with" hard feelings.

Learning to feel and *be with* your feelings requires patience and mindfulness. Think of your feelings as little children calling for your attention. They need to be heard, soothed, and comforted. Not pushed aside as if they—and you—don't matter. Your feelings *do* matter and are there to teach you something. For example, unexpressed anger may be teaching you to speak up for yourself, resentment may be helping you to set boundaries, and sadness may be guiding you to grieve the loss of the loving family you never had.

When you mute your feelings with food, you unintentionally deny yourself opportunities for growth that keep you from healing old wounds. Just as a crying baby needs to be soothed in their mother's loving arms, your feelings need that tender approach too. (You'll learn how to do this in chapter 6.)

Let's now look at another way to give your feelings the validation and attention they deserve.

Releasing Traumatic Secrets

There's a saying in Alcoholics Anonymous that teaches a powerful truth: "You're as sick as your secrets."

This doesn't only apply to someone with an alcohol problem. This applies to everyone. There's a difference between keeping an experience in your life private versus keeping it secret. If something is private, you generally share it with people you trust. You don't want everyone to know your business but feel comfortable telling your closest loved ones.

Secrets, however, can feel shame-inducing. Something seems so horrible or forbidden that it doesn't feel safe to share. You worry that people will judge you, blame you, or think you are "damaged goods." It's not unusual for people to hold secrets about the trauma they experienced, unless that trauma was "socially acceptable." For example, it's easier to share an early loss or that your parents divorced. These certainly are traumatic experiences and, depending on the circumstances, may be fraught with shame. But chances are, they're easier to mention than the trauma of abuse and neglect.

Especially during childhood, traumatic secrets take an emotional toll. Without a trusted adult to talk with—and sometimes *even with* trusted adults in their lives—children often feel too timid, afraid, or ashamed to disclose the trauma they're experiencing, especially when perpetrated by family members. Think about it: Parents have extreme power over their children. Kids do not tell on them. They're psychologically wired to not betray their family. They rarely divulge that their mother hits them or their father slurs his words after drinking beer. And whether the perpetrator is a family or nonfamily member, the shame of sexual abuse and fear of not being believed—or threatened if they tell—prevents them from disclosing that secret. Food softens the pain and isolation of not talking.

There certainly are situations where children do disclose that they're being harmed. This mostly occurs with adolescents who become somewhat less fearful than when they were younger. And when a perpetrator is not a close family member *and* the child or teen has strong family relationships, *and* they have not been threatened with harm to themselves or their family to stay silent, they may feel safe disclosing that someone is hurting them. But for children traumatized by a family member or someone who holds authority, such as a teacher, athletic coach, or religious leader, disclosing is difficult, if not impossible.

Child abuse is twofold: it's the traumatic experience itself coupled with the emotional heaviness of not expressing your feelings about it. This results in unprocessed fear that lives in your body and mind and, as you're learning, is why your body becomes easily dysregulated.

For example, Carol's brother sexually abused her for years. He told her he would go to jail if anyone found out. She couldn't bear feeling responsible for that—despite what was happening, she loved her big brother. She never told anyone until she started therapy as an adult. Carol not only was traumatized from being sexually abused but also experienced the added trauma from being unable to talk about it. Candy and cupcakes became her trusted friends.

Even if traumatic experiences are known within a family, the child's feelings may remain secret. For example, Carol's relatives knew her mother physically abused her, but no one intervened. She learned that keeping a smile on her face kept friends and teachers from asking if anything was wrong. What would she say if they asked? She hid her sadness and fear inside. Food helped her cope.

Holding the secret of childhood trauma—perhaps for decades—can make you sick physically, emotionally, and spiritually. The inner tension that comes from unprocessed traumatic secrets is part of the reason you may experience anxiety, sadness, and emptiness that triggers emotional eating. You'll learn more about unprocessed emotions and how to release them in chapter 6.

If you were able to disclose and process the trauma you experienced when you were a child, I'm happy for you. But if you weren't able to, it's not too late to release your secrets and their emotionally harmful effects.

Emotional intimacy comes from self-disclosure. When we share our innermost thoughts and feelings, we connect with people on a deep level. Secrets, however, create barriers between you and important people in your life. If you have been unable to tell anyone about the trauma you experienced as a child, it's understandable that you may feel emotional isolation and shame. When those hard feelings are triggered, food helps you cope.

Sharing the secret of childhood abuse or neglect with trusted people can help you relax inner tension, feel more emotionally connected, and offer you the promise of support. Maybe you've told some people about what happened to you. If so, congratulate yourself for taking this step.

If you have never told anyone about the abuse you experienced as a child, will you consider doing so? You may be thinking, *No way. I can't do that. I'm too afraid of what people may think.* It's understandable that you may feel uncomfortable with this. Some of my clients never told their partners about early trauma until after they started therapy and with my encouragement. It *is* hard. I'm discussing this because emotional eating may feel easier to heal when the trauma you experienced is no longer a secret.

Sharing painful experiences before you feel ready would not be good for you. It's important to be thoughtful about it, so no pressure. Simply reflect on the idea. Take your time to think about whom you could tell and what it would mean to finally share this secret and no longer feel alone with it. Here are some suggestions and points to consider:

- Think of someone you know whom you trust and feel safe with. Perhaps this is your partner, friend, or family member. What would it be like to tell this person you were abused or neglected as a child? When you think of this person, recall times in the past you shared sensitive information and how they reacted. If they were compassionate with other difficult issues, chances are they will respond the same way this time.

- If a relative abused you, sharing this with someone in your family may be complicated. Is there a family member you trust who would be supportive no matter what?

- Does it seem possible to tell your significant other? Can you imagine it would bring you closer and explain some of your fear-based behaviors? Or do you worry that they'll feel hurt or angry that you hadn't told them before? Sometimes telling the closest people in our lives offers much-needed support. Other times it feels extra hard and is fraught with confusion. If telling your significant other feels too difficult, that's okay. It may be best to tell a therapist or friend first and decide later if you want to tell them. That's not a betrayal. It's taking care of yourself.

- If you can think of someone you want to tell, trust that the right moment will present itself. No need to force this. Let your intuition guide you.

Even when considering telling a trusted person about the trauma you experienced, saying the words can feel hard. Here are some suggestions.

You could start with, "There's something I want to tell you that's hard for me to talk about." Sometimes it's helpful to add the very thing you fear. For example, "But I'm afraid you'll think less of me," or "I'm afraid you'll wonder why I never told you before, so I hope you'll understand that this has been hard for me." Putting your fears up front gets them out of the way. Then you could say, "I had a tough childhood," or "I went through some difficult experiences growing up." You could then add, "I've never told anyone before and wanted you to know. I trust you, and I don't want to feel alone with this anymore." Depending on how the person responds, you decide if you want to say anything more. If you do, then continue sharing what you're comfortable with. If not, you could say, "You know, just saying this is a big step for me. Thanks for listening. Maybe we can talk more another time." This first conversation opens a door. You decide how far it goes.

If you don't feel comfortable sharing with people close to you right now, I encourage you to let your health care provider or gynecologist know that you experienced childhood trauma. Gynecological appointments in particular can be hard, even traumatic, for sexual abuse survivors. Many of my clients would either avoid making these appointments or experience anxiety beforehand. By letting your gynecologist know about your trauma history, they then may be extra patient with you.

Informing your health care providers about your history gives them important information to better offer you care. As mentioned earlier, the ACES study reveals a direct link between childhood trauma and later physical and mental health issues. Some providers ask on an intake form if patients experienced trauma. Answering this could be a starting point. Or, if you feel safe and comfortable with your provider, you could say, "There's something I want to tell you. It may be important for you to know that I experienced trauma as a child. I'm learning that this could have affected my stress level and health." They may have some resources to offer you. For example, they could refer you to a licensed mental health practitioner if you would like to start therapy.

Let's now move on to a third relaxation practice. As you're learning, the ability to calm your body and nervous system is an important skill to help you heal both childhood trauma and emotional eating. Along with diaphragmatic breathing, progressive muscle relaxation (PMR) is another practice that is especially helpful for trauma survivors to release tension from their bodies and muscles.

Progressive Muscle Relaxation

Physician and psychiatrist Edmund Jacobson developed PMR in the 1920s. PMR is a simple technique to calm your body. It involves tightening and relaxing different muscle groups. PMR helps you notice how your body feels when your muscles are tense and when they're relaxed. Recognizing this difference helps you develop interoceptive awareness of when your body feels stressed. Many of my clients didn't realize how much tension they were holding in their bodies until they learned PMR.

Speak with your health care provider before learning PMR if you have muscle pain, joint issues, or medical concerns that could be aggravated by this process.

The following is a shortened version of PMR. (You can download a longer audio version at http://www.newharbinger.com /51178.) Be sure to wear loose clothing. I suggest you first practice PMR sitting in a firm, comfortable chair. After you become familiar with the process, you can do this in a reclining position or lying down, whichever feels best for you.

Sitting in your chair, take several diaphragmatic breaths to settle yourself. Then, simply breathe in whatever way feels natural to you. To keep your breathing even and not strained during PMR, breathe in synchrony with tensing and relaxing each muscle: inhale as you tense a muscle and exhale as you release it.

We'll now move through the different parts of your body, starting from your face and moving to your shoulders, arms, torso, and down to your legs and feet. When directed to tighten the muscles, do so firmly but not so tightly as to strain yourself, and you'll tense and release each body area twice before moving on to the next area.

Begin by tightening the muscles in your face and forehead. You can do this by squinting your eyes and pressing your lips together. Hold the tension for a few seconds and notice what that feels like. Then, release the tension. Notice what the sense of release feels like. Repeat once more.

Then, shrug your shoulders up high and tight. Hold a few seconds while noticing the tension. Then release and relax your shoulders. Notice the difference between tension and relaxation. Repeat once more.

Then, moving onto your arms, extend your right arm, clench your fist, and tighten the muscles in your arm. Hold the tension for a moment and notice the sensations in your arm. Then release the tension and relax the arm and hand. Notice the sensations in your arm as it is relaxed. Repeat once more. Then repeat the process with your left arm.

Then, moving onto your torso, tighten the muscles in your chest and stomach to whatever degree feels comfortable. Remember not to strain yourself. Notice what the tension feels like. Then let go and relax. Notice the sensation of relaxation. Repeat the process.

Moving onto your legs, extend your right leg, flex your right foot, and tighten the muscles throughout your leg and foot. Hold for a moment and notice the sensation of tension. Then release the tightness, put the leg down, and notice the sensation of relaxation. Repeat this process once more with your right leg. Then repeat this process twice with your left leg and foot.

I suggest you practice PMR daily in the beginning. This way, you're not only giving your mind, body, and nervous system the benefits of relaxation, but you're also learning where in your body you hold the most tension. You then can focus only on those areas throughout the day.

Putting It All Together

We've covered a lot here. How are you doing? Reflecting on your early experiences with food and emotional eating and learning about the effect of trauma on your body may not feel easy, but it's important to see your emotional eating behaviors in the context of your early struggles. Everyone's behavior—including your own—makes sense when you learn their history and the burdens they carry. So be gentle with yourself. You've been doing the best you can.

Take time to reflect on whether you'd like to share with someone about the trauma you experienced. Perhaps you'd like to journal about this to gain clarity on what's best for you.

Do you need some self-compassion right now? You've done a great job reading through this material, and it may have felt unsettling. If you wish, get quiet, take a moment, and wrap your arms around yourself to give you—and your inner child—a warm hug. Giving yourself hugs can feel grounding and nurturing and offers you a simple self-loving gift when you feel triggered.

Next, we'll address what emotional eating looks and feels like when you have a history of trauma and how to notice your body's signs of hunger and fullness so you can become the attentive caretaker it needs you to be.

CHAPTER 2

Emotional Eating: Your Refuge and a Source of Pain

One of the challenges of healing emotional eating is giving up a habit that helps you. When you feel overwhelmed by strong emotion, food becomes your sanctuary from inner chaos. When you're focused on the food you're eating, you're less focused on what bothered you in the first place. Eventually, you calm down. But eating then becomes a source of pain: you become upset with yourself for eating, perhaps worry that this may add weight to your body and, especially if you've been yo-yo dieting for years, judge yourself as "bad." Beating yourself up for eating then gets in the way of healing because you're not addressing the underlying emotions you've numbed with food. (You'll learn more about how to process emotions in chapter 6.) Let's explore further how this pattern started and why emotional eating was, in fact, a resourceful way for you to cope.

For their optimal growth and development, children need to feel safe and secure and live carefree lives. They depend on their parents and caretakers to meet their basic needs for shelter, food, clothing, physical safety, and their emotional needs for human warmth, love, and comfort.

When children are emotionally distressed and receive comforting care and attention from a trusted adult, they internalize compassion and experience relief. The external support they receive helps them develop internal strength. They learn that feelings are natural, feelings come and go, and feelings are not to be feared. When adults consistently offer children support, they're teaching the child how to self-soothe. For example, simply hearing reassuring words, such as, "I know you're sad, sweetie. It will be okay," gives children the model of reassuring words that becomes their own self-talk. For example, "It will be okay" becomes "I'm okay." Receiving comfort is crucial so children can develop into adults who feel worthy to give themselves good care.

When their needs are met, children generally can thrive emotionally, spiritually, and physically despite typical family and life stressors. When they go to sleep at night, they feel safe in their parents' loving care. Their bodies and nervous systems can relax.

Early soothing gives children the experience of relief; the absence of soothing leaves children feeling desperate. They're alone with hard feelings and don't experience comfort when sad or scared. They learn that feelings are hard to bear and need to be pushed away. They don't learn the foundational tools for healthy self-care. (You'll learn more about how children cope with trauma in chapter 3.)

When children are traumatized and abused—particularly when the abuser is a family member they live with—they cannot feel safe. While some of their basic needs may be met, their world is dangerous because the threat of emotional, physical, or sexual danger exists and they do not receive help. This threat may be within the child's home, a relative or neighbor's house, school, church, camp, sports activities, dance class, neighborhood streets, and so on. When the child is unable to disclose the harm they're experiencing and it continues (or they disclose and it continues anyway), they suffer inescapable stress and trauma. Their bodies cannot relax.

At thirty-five, Todd still has a hard time relaxing. Raised by an alcoholic mother and physically abusive father, he felt alone and frightened much of his childhood. He breathed sighs of momentary relief when his father went to work and was constantly worried about his mother's daily drinking.

His parents not only couldn't comfort Todd, but they also were the source of his distress. Stealing money from his mother's purse to buy candy at the corner store became his reliable source of support. When he first started therapy, finding comfort in food was the only way Todd knew how to cope.

Even when home life is physically safe, it may be bereft of emotional support. For example, Serena was ten years old when her mother died suddenly in a car accident. Her grieving father didn't know how to care for Serena and her three younger siblings, so Aunt Vicky stepped in to help. She tended to the family's physical needs but didn't know how to handle emotional needs. No one talked to Serena about her mother or soothed her sadness and grief. No one knew that Serena developed anxiety about losing her father and aunt too. They thought she was hyperactive. Serena's father and aunt couldn't offer her relief. Sweets from the pantry helped Serena ease her fear and anxious body. At forty-five, she still struggled with panic and abandonment fears. Food was her go-to source of comfort and emotional stability.

A traumatized child or teen may not even be aware of feeling stressed when they seek food. They just know that eating candy, cookies, and other foods helps them feel better. The same may apply to you when you mindlessly eat for no apparent reason. Given the trauma you experienced, it's understandable. You have your reasons. So stop judging yourself, okay?

Five Differences Between Emotional and Physical Hunger

We'll now discuss what emotional eating looks and feels like when you have a history of trauma by identifying five differences between emotional hunger and physical hunger. These differences are adapted from the eight traits of emotional hunger published in Constant Craving: What Your Food Cravings Mean and How to Overcome Them, by Doreen Virtue, PhD (1995, 30–31). Knowledge of these differences helps you develop conscious awareness and nonjudgmental acceptance of behaviors that feel out of your control.

Use this framework to reflect on your current eating habits and to inform you as you develop new ones. You may find it helpful to use your journal and write down whatever thoughts and feelings emerge as you read these. I'll offer some prompts to guide you. Some of the questions may seem similar, but when you reflect on your eating behavior in slightly different ways, you can gain new insights.

1. Emotional hunger occurs in response to your feelings and trauma-based sensations in your body. Physical hunger occurs because your body needs fuel. With emotional hunger, any feeling that is difficult to regulate and causes unsettling sensations in your body may trigger the urge to eat. This includes painful feelings and, while it may sound counterintuitive, uplifting ones too. For example, you feel lonely at night and eat cookies for comfort. You feel anxious about finances and eat a bag of chips to relieve the stress. Or, you feel excited about booking a vacation with friends and eat a bowl of ice cream after feeling full from dinner. Of course, there's nothing wrong with eating ice cream. What I'm referring to is a pattern of eating behavior that pushes away hard feelings—loneliness, fear—that need your compassionate attention or dampens joyful feelings if you then beat yourself up for eating.

Now here's the thing. It's actually not the feelings themselves that prompt the urge to eat; it's the inability to let yourself *feel and be with your feelings* without adding food to the mix. It may be easier for you to understand why you eat when feeling stressed or overwhelmed, but *any* feeling can trigger the urge to eat. When uplifting emotions lead to eating, it's sometimes due to feeling unsettled, often unconsciously, with a happy state. This isn't unusual for people who experienced early trauma. When your default state is sadness, fear, or unworthiness, positive feelings themselves can be unsettling. Deep inside, you may feel nondeserving or don't trust that the feeling is real or will last, which may elicit disquieting sensations in your body on a level you're not even aware of.

Either way, with painful or uplifting feelings, you're finding it impossible to simply *feel* without needing to do anything else. For some people, any emotion can trigger the urge to eat; for others, it's mostly painful ones. And sometimes, you simply don't know why.

In contrast to emotional hunger, physical hunger is biologically based. When you haven't eaten in a while, your body communicates it needs food with a rumbling in your belly, light-headed feeling, or difficulty concentrating. You may feel irritable or "hangry." When you're attuned to your body's needs and have developed greater interoceptive awareness, you don't let yourself get overly hungry. For example, if it's been several hours since you ate a meal, you feel a little hungry and eat to keep your body balanced and well nourished.

Eating to assuage physical hunger has nothing to do with your mood, so you feel neutral about eating and the food you choose. (This may feel complicated, however, if you designate some foods as forbidden due to years of restrictive dieting. You'll learn more about making peace with food in chapter 7.)

JOURNAL PROMPTS: *Notice why you're eating.*

- Think of the last time you ate due to feeling stressed or overwhelmed. What emotion or situation triggered the urge to eat? How did you and your body feel after eating? Simply write down your experience without judgment.

- Think of a time you ate in response to feeling excited or happy. Did you feel neutral about eating? Or, did you feel upset with yourself? If so, how did being upset affect the excitement you initially felt?

- Think of a time you noticed signs of physical hunger and ate something to honor your body's need for fuel, with no guilt. What was that experience like? If it's hard to recall a time of being connected with your body this way, that's okay. We'll be addressing below how to notice your body's signs of hunger and fullness.

After journaling, breathe and write this: "I accept myself and know that I'm doing the best I can."

2. Emotional hunger tends to come on suddenly. Physical hunger emerges gradually. When your emotions drive your craving, the impulse to eat can feel sudden, intense, and urgent. You confuse an emotional need with a physical one. It's not about food, but food is the only thing on your mind. If you're in a situation where you can't access food in the moment, you obsess about what and when you'll eat.

For example, you had an argument with your partner and suddenly feel the urge to eat, so you grab something from the fridge even though you had lunch an hour ago. Your body isn't hungry, but it *is* responding to your emotional state. It's hard to tolerate your body's sensations of stress, and you know that food will help you feel better.

There are situations, however, when emotional hunger doesn't only come on suddenly but lingers chronically in your mind and heart. You may be feeling so despondent that turning to food on a regular basis is your way of self-medicating. Mealtimes don't only meet a biological need; they're opportunities for self-soothing. It's hard to know when your body is full because your heart feels empty. Eating becomes a habit that helps you get through the day.

In contrast to emotional hunger, with physical hunger, the sensations in your body develop over time. If you're attuned to your body's needs, you sense the early signs that your body needs food. For example, you notice rumbling or a slight emptiness in your stomach. You feel in charge of these early cues. Food is something you begin to desire, but it can wait until you feel ready to eat. If you're unable to access food, these sensations intensify until you're able to give your body the fuel it needs. (Sometimes, however, physical hunger does come on suddenly due to blood sugar instability. Talk with your health care provider to see if this applies to you.)

JOURNAL PROMPTS: *Notice the timing of eating.*

- Think of a time when the urge to eat came on suddenly (unrelated to a medical issue). What did you eat, and what was the situation that triggered you?

- Think of a time you noticed your body's physical hunger signs slowly developing. What were those signs, and how did you respond? How often do you give your body food without emotions dictating what or how much you eat? You may be so focused on eating for emotional reasons that you don't acknowledge the times you honor your body's need for fuel alone, and I bet those times are there too. (If you can't think of a time right now, that's okay. You're learning.)

3. With emotional hunger, you crave certain foods. With physical hunger, you're open to many options.

When you eat for emotional reasons, you tend to want specific foods, often ones that are high fat, sugary, or salty. You've discovered that eating certain foods calms you, so you're not open to other options. You probably have your go-to foods that help you feel better. Some of my clients' comfort foods are ice cream, cookies, chips, french fries, cheeseburgers, pasta, and bread. I bet you can relate.

I want to emphasize that there is nothing "wrong" with these, or any, foods. When people eat for emotional reasons, some foods work better than others to soothe those hard feelings. This isn't about judging food as "good" or "bad" or judging yourself as "good" or "bad" for eating or not eating them. Turning to these foods has nothing to do with poor judgment or a lack of willpower. You're just trying to help yourself feel better.

In contrast to emotional hunger, when you're physically hungry, you still may have your preferences but are open to many choices. For example, you may desire a ham-and-cheese sandwich for lunch, but if that's not available, even raw carrots and celery will look appealing to your rumbling stomach. (Nothing against carrots and celery, by the way.) You eat enough of whatever food is available, and even if not your preferred food, you feel satisfied because your body's need for fuel was met and you're not trying to meet an emotional need.

JOURNAL PROMPTS: *Notice what you enjoy eating.*

- What are your go-to foods when you feel upset? How do you feel emotionally and in your body after eating them at those times?

- What are your favorite foods generally? How do you feel when you eat them and are not triggered by emotional hunger?

4. Emotional hunger doesn't notice signs of physiological fullness. With physical hunger only, you stop eating when full. Emotional hunger can lead to mindless eating. You keep eating until you become numb to the feeling that triggered the impulse to eat. You're not attuned to your body because you're satisfying an emotional need not a physical one. Your body may be saying, "I'm full now, you can stop eating," but you don't notice or heed that message because your mind is saying, "I can't tolerate these hard feelings. I need to keep eating to stop feeling this way." The grip of emotional hunger and nervous system dysregulation override your ability to notice your body telling you it's full.

In contrast, when you eat because you're physically hungry (and emotional eating is no longer a challenge), you know when you're ready to stop eating. You feel attuned to your body's needs and notice the increasing sensations of fullness. You make a conscious choice to stop when your body feels satisfied and reasonably full.

JOURNAL PROMPTS: *Notice how your body feels after eating.*

- Think of a time you ate to the point of physical discomfort. What and how much did you eat? How did your body feel? Was it stuffed, lethargic, nauseous? How much food would have been enough to satisfy your body? If you're not sure, that's okay. Simply reflecting on the question helps you consider how much food is "enough."

- Think of a time you ate exactly what your body needed and felt physically satisfied. How did you and your body feel afterward? What was it like to meet your body's need for fuel only and not eat for emotional reasons? Again, if you can't think of a time, that's fine. You're just not there *yet*.

5. Emotional eating often induces feelings of guilt or shame. Eating to satisfy physical hunger only does not. Emotional eating episodes perpetuate a cycle of self-blame. You eat because you're upset or to enhance an uplifting feeling. You feel better *at first* because food numbs your hard feelings and accentuates the uplifting ones. But then, you feel guilt and shame for eating. What has been a source of refuge from painful emotions, or a habit in response to *any* strong feeling, then becomes a source of pain.

Guilt and shame are core issues for many trauma survivors, especially abuse victims. When eating triggers these feelings, it's not only about the food. The guilt and shame for emotional eating bring to the surface the guilt and shame *that already are inside of you.* Your intention with eating is to feel better, but instead you get caught in a cycle of reexperiencing old pain. This compounding effect makes these feelings especially powerful and hard to bear. You're not only feeling guilt and shame for eating, although that's what you're focusing on. You're actually feeling trauma-based guilt and shame that have been held in your body and subconscious mind from earlier in your life. Even though a trauma may have happened a long time ago, if your feelings weren't acknowledged and addressed, they continue to live inside you. I want to reassure you that once you begin to heal past trauma, the underlying guilt and shame, and other trauma-based feelings, won't be as easily triggered or as intense. In chapters 5 and 6, you'll learn how to process trauma-based beliefs and feelings. For now, just know that experiencing guilt and shame is not unusual for trauma survivors, you're not alone, and congratulate yourself for having the confidence to travel this journey.

In contrast to emotional eating, when you eat to satisfy physical hunger only, your body feels nourished and you feel content. You know that eating fulfills a physical need and no longer is enmeshed with feeding an emotional one. Even when you eat a favorite food to the point that your body feels uncomfortably full, you don't beat yourself up. You accept you enjoyed your favorite meal to excess and let it go. As you heal trauma-based feelings, you'll notice a lessening, and perhaps elimination, of guilt, shame, and self-judgment—no matter what or how much you ate.

JOURNAL PROMPTS: *Notice how you feel after eating.*

- Write about a time you felt guilt or shame for eating. After journaling, add: "I am releasing shame and guilt from my mind, heart, and body."

- Write about a neutral eating experience. You gave your body the food it needed with no judgment. How common is this, and what was it like for you?

Another reason why some trauma survivors use food as sanctuary relates to feeling vulnerable in their body. As mentioned earlier, this book is not about weight loss. It is possible, however, that some people may release weight as they heal emotional eating and become attuned to their body's needs. Additionally, for some people, especially sexual abuse survivors, added weight may have developed as a form of emotional and physical protection from sexual maltreatment or other aggression. Releasing weight then may feel triggering because it can elicit feelings of vulnerability as that protection fades. I want to underscore that this does not apply to all sexual abuse survivors nor are all sexual abuse survivors of a higher weight. But for some people, these fears are real. If this applies to you, it is possible that you may feel a disquieting nervousness if you start to release weight. Emotional eating understandably then helps you feel safe. The dynamic I'm describing is not unusual, and you're not alone. I hope my mentioning this helps you feel validated with behaviors and reactions that may feel confusing to you.

If releasing weight triggers fear and vulnerability, or if traumatic memories or flashbacks overwhelm you or lead you to feeling unsafe with yourself, it's important to seek support from a licensed mental health practitioner. Healing emotional eating coupled with a history of trauma can be a hard road. Feeling vulnerable in your body and intrusive traumatic memories make it especially difficult. But with professional help, you'll have a place to safely process and move through these issues. So please get the support you need and don't travel this journey alone, okay? (I offer psychotherapy resources later in this book.)

Now that you've learned the differences between emotional hunger and physical hunger, let's look at how your body tells you when it is hungry and full.

Learn Your Body's Hunger and Fullness Signals

As you heal emotional eating and become attuned to your body, it's important to learn how your body lets you know when it needs food and when it's had enough. While trauma and a dysregulated nervous system can get in the way of noticing these signs, your body, nevertheless, is still communicating with you. Practicing diaphragmatic breathing and progressive muscle relaxation (PMR) will help quiet your nervous system, which is a first step to help you notice your body's hunger and fullness signals. The next thing you do is start paying attention.

Let's begin by identifying your body's signs of hunger and fullness.

Hunger sensations include:

an empty feeling in the stomach

stomach pangs or growling

light-headedness, headache, shakiness

low energy or fatigue

irritability

difficulty concentrating.

Can you relate to these? What other ways does your body tell you it needs food?

Fullness sensations include:

the absence of growling stomach as appetite is curbed

comfortable physical satisfaction

an uncomfortable fullness in the stomach

feeling stuffed to the point of discomfort

being in a "food coma," which is a state of lethargy, mental fogginess, and emotional numbness.

Can you relate to these? What other ways does your body tell you when it is full?

When your emotions dictate your eating habits, a full stomach doesn't necessarily stop you from eating. Nevertheless, noticing your body's hunger and fullness cues is an essential step to help you heal emotional eating and feel more connected to your body.

Here's a handy barometer to gauge and identify your body's signs of hunger, fullness, and satisfaction adapted from *The Intuitive Eating Workbook: Ten Principles for Nourishing a Healthy Relationship with Food*, by Evelyn Tribole and Elyse Resch (2017). (You can download a PDF version here: http://www.newharbinger.com/51178.)

Hunger-Fullness Scale

1. Starving. Feel light-headed and shaky.

2. Very hungry. Hard to concentrate. "Hangry."

3. Hungry and ready to eat.

4. Not hungry yet, but beginning to feel hungry.

5. Neutral. Neither hungry nor full.

6. Comfortably full and satisfied.

7. Very full. Feel a little uncomfortable.

8. Uncomfortably full. Clothes feel tight around waist.

9. Very uncomfortably full. Almost feel sick.

10. Overly full. Stuffed and numb. In a "food coma."

Write the scale in your phone or on small cards to keep with you during the day. You could put one in your purse, desk drawer at work, or in your kitchen—wherever you think having it accessible will help.

Take a moment right now to notice your body's hunger-fullness signs. As you're learning, calming your body helps you develop interoceptive awareness, so start by taking a few diaphragmatic breaths. Then, get quiet and with eyes open or closed, direct your attention to your body, especially in the area of your torso and head. Notice the sensations you experience. Then, review the scale to see what words describe how satisfied, hungry, or full you feel. What number best matches how your body feels? If you can't tell right now, that's okay because this is a skill you can learn.

One way to develop this skill is to practice noticing your body's hunger-fullness signs for a set number of days. For example, designate two or three days (or perhaps a week) to check in with your body every one, two, or three hours, or whatever timeframe best suits your schedule. Using the directions above, pause, breathe, settle yourself, and notice how your body feels based on the scale. Keep a notebook handy to record the number and time of day, as this gives you valuable information to learn your body's hunger-fullness patterns. Then do your best to honor what your body is telling you.

After you've practiced, make it a habit to review the scale several times each day. Especially before, during, and after each meal, rate your hunger-fullness level. The goal is to stay within the three and six zones of the scale. Sometimes you'll achieve this, and sometimes you won't. That's okay. Life gets in the way for everyone at times. The most important thing is to practice. At some point, you won't need an external scale to review because you will have internalized how to interpret your body's signs. But that takes time, so have patience.

This attentive focus helps you become attuned to your body's needs. Think of a devoted mother who is learning how to care for her newborn baby. She listens and pays attention to the nuance of her baby's cries, smiles, eating, and sleep habits. This gives her information so she can best care for her child's needs. Does the baby's cry mean she's hungry, needs to be changed, or is tired? After a while, an attentive mother learns how her baby communicates with her. Using the hunger-fullness scale in an intentional, observant way helps you too become a nurturing and devoted caretaker for your body.

When you eat for emotional reasons, physical fullness can feel so skewed and unreliable that it's easy to detach from what your body truly needs. This detachment applies not only to overeating but also to not eating enough. That's why it's not unusual for people who emotionally eat to also disregard their body's legitimate need for fuel. Using the hunger-fullness scale will help.

For example, Tasara's habit was to skip lunch during her workday because "I'm not hungry." At night, however, she tended to eat dinner to the point of feeling uncomfortably full. Later in the evening, she'd eat again. She wasn't always emotionally eating—she sometimes was famished and needed food—but detachment from her body made it difficult to notice its signals. After she practiced using the hunger-fullness scale, she noticed feeling hungry during the day. She was so used to disregarding her body's needs that she created an untrue reality. It wasn't that she wasn't hungry at lunchtime. It was that she wasn't paying attention.

Once Tasara started paying attention, she learned her body needed fuel around 11:30 a.m. and again at 3:30 p.m. She began bringing a healthy lunch and nutritious snacks to eat on her break. Tasara then wasn't famished when she got home after work, so she could eat comfortably at dinner. Like a mother who senses the difference between her baby's cries for food and needing to be held, becoming attuned to hunger-fullness signs helped Tasara develop a more connected relationship with her body. (You'll learn more about deepening your relationship with your body in chapter 4.)

Putting It All Together

How are you doing? What was it like to reflect on using food as refuge from trauma and pain? That's a lot to take in, so if it feels overwhelming, it's understandable. Pause and breathe.

What was it like to learn the differences between emotional hunger and physical hunger and how to use the hunger-fullness scale? Learning about new ways of approaching food, eating, and listening to your body may feel daunting. That often happens when we're standing at the border from where we are and looking at where we want to go. We wonder, *How will I ever get there?* Change *can* feel daunting. That's normal. So be gentle with yourself and trust that you were drawn to this book because a part of you—your Wise Self part—knows you have what it takes.

Perhaps you'd like to pause and journal about your insights. You're doing a great job sticking with this. These aren't easy topics to navigate, so congratulate yourself for digging deep this way. Remember to breathe diaphragmatically, visit your peaceful place, and use progressive muscle relaxation to feel calm and settled as necessary. When you're ready, continue to chapter 3, where you'll learn more about how early trauma affected your brain and nervous system. I'll also teach you a beautiful self-compassion practice that will help you and your body feel safe and secure.

CHAPTER 3

Calm Your Anxious Brain

Childhood traumatic stress, especially when chronic and inescapable, shapes the child's developing brain chemistry so that the nervous system remains stuck in trauma. The chronic activation of the amygdala's fight-flight-freeze response and release of the stress hormones cortisol and adrenaline can lead to a dysregulated nervous system and hypersensitivity to even mild forms of stress later in life.

What exactly is your nervous system? Simply put, your brain is the command center, and via a network of nerves throughout your body, it controls every aspect of your health and functioning, including your thoughts, emotions, memory, senses, movements, digestion, sleep, and breathing. Early trauma can affect your brain in such a way that this network of nerves keeps the trauma alive. Have you heard the phrase "our issues are in our tissues"? That's what it refers to. It's as if your body is a time capsule holding the experience of early trauma. When triggered, you may feel the sensation of fear in your body, a sinking feeling in your gut, or disorientation of awareness. Self-soothing and regulation strategies, like diaphragmatic breathing, peaceful place imagery, and progressive muscle relaxation will help in those moments. (You'll learn more strategies later in this book too.) But when you don't know how to regulate your dysregulated body, it's understandable that you may reach for food to ground yourself.

Food *is* a quick fix. Those trauma-based sensations in your body are hard to deal with, and you're just trying to find relief. But when using food is your primary coping tool, it doesn't help you get to the root cause of your body's dysregulation. It may calm your body in the moment but doesn't work in the long run.

Let's look further at how early trauma affects the nervous system.

When we perceive a threat, our body needs that heightened state of alertness—the fight-flight-freeze response—for our survival. When the threat is gone, however, our body needs to recover. As adults, we have control over helping our body recover from stress, and I show you ways to do that throughout this book. But for children, ongoing and inescapable abuse and trauma leave no room for the child's body to recover from chronic stress. Without this recovery, the child's stress response system becomes compromised. Many traumatized children then move into adulthood with an impaired ability to respond to stress or feel at peace in their body. This is why you may feel vulnerable to emotional eating triggers. It's not your fault, and it's not a weakness; it's about how your brain and nervous system adapted to early trauma.

If you experienced trauma as an adult and not in childhood, most likely your nervous system had a chance to recover because you have resources available that helpless children don't have. Nevertheless, and depending on the trauma you experienced, your nervous system may respond in a heightened way when you feel even slightly threatened. The grounding and self-calming suggestions in this book will help you too.

Caregivers and Childhood Stress

To emotionally survive, traumatized and abused children need to find a way to not feel burdened by the conscious awareness of a scary life. They may appear carefree, but that's on the surface. On a deeper level, they're pushing away their fears and feelings into their subconscious mind. This is an automatic response, the mind's way of helping children bear the unbearable. They then can play video games, play soccer, and laugh with family and friends, all the while holding inside fear and scary secrets.

But scary secrets take a toll. Pain that cannot be spoken—and abuse that doesn't stop—leaves the child in a state of chronic fear and stress. As you learned above, stress that cannot be released from the body disrupts the body's natural ability to restore itself.

Caregivers play a critical role in shaping the child's developing brain and stress response. That's because children are dependent upon their caregivers for support and protection. When soothed by caregivers, children learn how to soothe themselves. When their caretakers lovingly care for them, they learn how to treat themselves with loving self-care. Caregivers, therefore, can help regulate and calm the child's stress response or, as in abusive and neglectful families, routinely activate it. Emotional eating, and other compulsive behaviors, often stems from children and adolescents never having received care and comfort in response to the traumatic stress they were enduring.

Let's look at how the stress response works when a child is scared and lives with caretakers who comfort them:

Ten-year-old Suzie awakens to the boom of thunder. Startled and scared, her stress response gets triggered, and she lies in bed frozen. Her brain releases the stress hormones cortisol and adrenaline. Her muscles tense, her heart starts pounding, and her breathing becomes rapid and shallow. She's hyperalert, with eyes wide open.

Her body's natural stress response prepares Suzie to fight or flee so she can take action to protect herself. She runs into her parents' bedroom. Her parents reassure her, telling Suzie that it's just a storm, thunder can't hurt her, and everything is okay. She calms down. Her heart stops pounding. Her muscles and body relax. Suzie breathes easily. Her mother walks her back to her bedroom and stays with Suzie, rubbing her back after tucking her in. Suzie falls asleep feeling calm, safe, and loved.

Suzie's body responded the way it was supposed to. Her mind perceived a threat (the sound of thunder), and her body's stress response (fight-flight-freeze) kicked into survival mode. Suzie fled to her parents.

Once comforted, Suzie stopped feeling scared and calmed down. The stress hormones eventually stopped coursing through her body because she had safe, comforting adults to help her nervous system feel soothed and reassured. Her parents' loving attentiveness in the face of fear not only helped Suzy calm her body, but it also nurtured the belief that she was worthy of love and protection. Repeated experiences of caring attention give Suzy the emotional foundation necessary for developing self-soothing and healthy self-care skills as an adult.

But what if the threat isn't simply a thunderstorm?

What if the threat is a person?

And what if that person *also* is someone the child depends on?

What if the threat never goes away?

Let's look at how Krystal's nervous system reacts to stress. Ten-year-old Krystal awakens to the boom of thunder. Her stress response gets triggered, and her body freezes. Feeling scared, her brain releases cortisol and adrenaline. Her heart starts pounding. She runs into her parents' bedroom. Her father is passed out from drinking too much beer. In a hushed, angry tone, her mother tells her to go back to sleep. "It's just thunder," she says. "Don't be a baby. And don't you wake your father." Grabbing Krystal by the arm, she pulls her back into her bedroom and says, "Get into that bed. You know you're not supposed to get out of your room. Wait till I tell your father. He'll give you something to cry about." "I'm sorry, Mommy, I'm sorry. I won't do that again. I won't, I won't," said Krystal, sobbing. Krystal's body fills with fear and shame and never fully recovers from being on high alert. Her stress response finds no comforting release, so the levels of cortisol and adrenaline in her body remain high. Krystal's father uses his belt to punish her, so she fears what will happen in the morning. Alone and scared, Krystal cries herself to sleep holding a pillow over her head to block out the thunder. Because she lives with inescapable threats—her parents—Krystal's body can never fully recover. She cannot internalize how to self-soothe because she is not soothed by her parents. Her developing self-care abilities are compromised. Food, especially cookies she sneaks from the kitchen pantry, become her sanctuary and trusted friends because they help her feel safe. When she eats, her empty heart feels full and her anxious body calms down.

Like many abusive and neglectful parents, Krystal's parents also can be loving and kind. But when they're most likely affected by their own early and unhealed trauma and their default way of coping with stress and addictions is to lash out at Krystal with harsh words or physical abuse, they're creating, often unintentionally, a toxic home environment. Such chronic, unpredictable behavior adds another level of stress and confusion for their precious child.

For many of my clients, the experience of childhood fear without comfort was common. Even if Krystal's home experience is different from yours, and maybe you didn't use food to cope until you were older, I wonder if you can relate. If reading this is triggering for you, take a moment to pause. It's okay. Breathe. Put the book down. Write in your journal. Do whatever you need to ground yourself.

For children who are bullied, abused, and otherwise traumatized by someone they do not live with and it's never disclosed (or it's disclosed but not stopped), their bodies can relax within the safety of their immediate family. But they hold inside the knowledge that the offender—grandfather, grandmother, uncle, aunt, family friend, teacher, coach, priest, camp counselor, neighbor—can still hurt them. They never can feel completely at peace.

How Traumatized Children Manage the Stress Response

Thus far, you've learned how the amygdala in the brain activates the fight-flight-freeze response when faced with a threat. There's a fourth trauma response called fawn, a term coined by Pete Walker (2013), author of *Complex PTSD: From Surviving to Thriving: A Guide and Map for Recovering from Childhood Trauma*, that refers to people-pleasing and appeasing behaviors. In contrast to the amygdala's physiological response, fawn responses are behavioral adaptations to chronic stress that the child (and later adult) uses to avoid conflict or punishment, emotional abandonment, and to gain approval.

All four are more than stress responses. They're *survival strategies*. Let's look more closely at how children manage these four ways their brains respond to stress.

Fight Response

Fighting back to escape abuse is not an option for a child. They're either physically unable or vulnerable to the person or stronger child holding power over them. It's simply not safe or possible to fight back. When the child becomes a teenager, they may try to fight back. For those too young, afraid, or trapped, however, their stress response gets activated during the trauma, but there is no escape by fighting. Stress hormones course through the body with no means to release and recover. As discussed above, this can lead to a dysregulated nervous system.

Flight Response

The most effective response in any threatening situation is to flee, if one can. But in the same way an abused child or teen rarely can fight back, they also rarely can flee. Until a child or teen feels safe to tell a trusted adult about the abuse they're experiencing and they're protected, or they run away from a dangerous home situation, they cannot flee from inescapable stress and trauma. Fear activates their stress response, but their body cannot release it by fleeing.

In the example above, Suzie perceived a threat when she heard thunder. She fled to her parents' room where she experienced the reassurance she needed for her body to recover from the stress response. Krystal, however, tried to flee and seek comfort from her parents. But the people she sought for help were instead threatening. Her body could not recover, so the stress hormones stayed activated in her body.

Freeze Response

You're probably familiar with the freeze response as it applies to animals in the wild. When they feel threatened, some animals play dead. Their body freezes as they hope the predator doesn't see them and moves on.

The freeze response is commonly used with abused children, especially sexually abused children. Because they rarely can fight or flee, children may freeze by tightening their bodies and staying still or pretending to be asleep if in their beds. Some sexually abused children freeze and emotionally detach from their bodies by using the psychological defense mechanism called dissociation (you'll learn more about dissociation below). For example, Anna, a twenty-eight-year-old married mother of two, remembers how she dissociated and froze her body when her stepfather would sexually abuse her.

During the abuse, Anna would stare at the flowers on her bedroom wallpaper. She counted the purple petals, hoping the touching would stop by the time she reached one hundred. When it didn't stop, Anna would keep counting. "I think I hypnotized myself," she said, "sending my mind to some faraway place, away from my body while he did those things to me."

By freezing and keeping her mind laser-focused on the wallpaper, Anna emotionally disconnected from her body. Stress hormones filled her body each time, and especially because the sexual abuse was secret, no one helped Anna and her nervous system recover.

Children, especially traumatized children, are hypersensitive to their parents' or caretakers' moods and have fine-tuned the skill of recognizing danger. They may instinctively tense and freeze their body when they see an angry look on their mother's face or their stepfather returns home from the bar slurring his words. Freezing as a stress response helps the child stay under the radar, although they still may not escape their parents' wrath.

Fawn Response

As a conditioned behavioral response to inescapable stress, fawn refers to pleasing others to gain approval. (Think of what it means to fawn over someone.) The fawn adaptation is most often linked with childhood interpersonal trauma where the child has been abused or neglected by a parent or significant caretaker to whom they're deeply attached. Some abused children cope by becoming overcompliant and eager to please the adults around them, especially the adults they most fear—and love. For instance, Krystal, in the example above, desperately apologized to her mother for running into her parents' bedroom after feeling afraid. Most children will do whatever they can to avoid punishment and emotional abandonment. Fawning helps them try to gain approval and acceptance. It also conditions children to develop into adults who accept unacceptable behaviors, have difficulty setting boundaries and saying no, and who use people-pleasing behaviors to avoid conflict and rejection. If you use these fawning behaviors, you probably know how they're strong emotional eating triggers. Nothing sends you to the pantry faster than the resentment that comes from putting other people's needs above your own and doing something you don't want to do.

Now that you've learned how children respond and adapt to chronic stress, let's look at how, without intervention, these experiences can result in traumatic stress disorder symptoms in both childhood and adulthood.

The Difference Between PTSD and C-PTSD

Many people use the term post-traumatic stress disorder (PTSD) and developmental or complex post-traumatic stress disorder (C-PTSD) interchangeably. While they are similar, there are some important differences.

PTSD is generally used to describe a set of physiological and psychological symptoms stemming from a one-time or fairly short-lived trauma. For example, the trauma could be a sudden death, physical or sexual assault, or witnessing a violent act or accident. C-PTSD refers to physiological and psychological symptoms most often stemming from *chronic* abuse and trauma, especially during the formative childhood years. The specific trauma also could be a one-time event. But if the child didn't have the support they needed to process the trauma and it stays emotionally buried, a diagnosis of later C-PTSD may apply. For example, if a child witnessed their mother being attacked by her partner, their parent died, or they were injured in a car accident and no one talked with the child about what they experienced or offered ongoing emotional help, the internalized fear and overwhelm can affect development and cause C-PTSD symptoms. Racial trauma and societal violence also can cause C-PTSD because the child experiences a chronic lack of safety and protection in their wider world. Because childhood trauma affects psychological development, I'll be focusing on C-PTSD rather than PTSD.

Symptoms of C-PTSD

Think of C-PTSD on a continuum. At one end are "intrusive" responses, and on the other end are "numbing" or "avoidant" responses. These apply to children, adolescents, and adults. When you experience these, your body and emotions feel dysregulated and ungrounded. All can be emotional eating triggers in an attempt to cope with feeling overwhelmed. As you read the following list, notice which ones apply to you.

INTRUSIVE SYMPTOMS

Intrusive symptoms impact your mind and body in overt, observable ways. They include:

Hyperarousal: You often feel on edge or jumpy. It's hard for your body to relax.

Hypervigilance: You're mentally "on guard" and alert for danger, even in safe situations.

Startle response: When you hear an unexpected sound, you startle easily or feel frightened. Your body may suddenly lurch.

Memory flooding: You have intrusive thoughts and memories about early trauma or flashbacks where you feel you're reliving a traumatic event.

Sleep problems: These range from difficulty falling asleep, staying asleep, and early awakening, to nightmares (a scary dream) or night terrors (displaying signs of fear, such as screaming, that others hear but you don't recall).

Mood instability: You have angry outbursts, feel irritable and frustrated much of the time, or vacillate between elation and despair.

Anxiety and panic: You experience chronic fear and worry in your mind and fear-based symptoms in your body (increased heart rate, muscle tightness, head tension). You sometimes experience intense and acute anxiety or panic attacks, with no clear trigger.

NUMBING SYMPTOMS

Numbing, or avoidant, symptoms impact you in a less overt, yet equally debilitating way. These include:

Constricted affect: You feel emotionally numb or empty. You display a limited range of emotion. While you laugh and smile at times, your typical facial expression is flat.

Underlying depression: While it may not get in the way of living your life (as with a more severe clinical depression), a chronic state of underlying depression may feel "normal" because you've felt this way for so long. You may not be aware that you look sad much of the time.

Limited emotional intimacy: You have a hard time expressing your emotions and tend not to share personal information with others. Since emotional intimacy depends on self-disclosure, you have a hard time feeling close to people.

Avoidance: You may avoid talking about your feelings and the trauma you experienced or minimize its impact. Childhood memories may be vague or hazy.

Dissociation: You feel psychologically disconnected from yourself and the world. During early trauma, dissociation creates a barrier that helps soften the impact so that the child shuts down emotionally, enters an altered state of consciousness, and may stop feeling what's happening in their body. Some trauma survivors describe looking down on themselves from the ceiling during episodes of physical or sexual abuse. Especially with chronic childhood trauma, dissociative states can continue into adulthood.

Think of dissociation on a continuum. We all dissociate at times, entering an altered state of consciousness in mild ways. For example, you're dissociating when engrossed in a book and don't notice someone entering the room or you're driving on the highway thinking about your to-do list and miss your exit. Your mind is laser-focused on one thing—your book, tasks—so your perception narrows. We all experience these moments, and they do not necessarily compromise our functioning or the connection we feel with our bodies.

When used as a psychological defense mechanism, however, dissociation sometimes can be extreme. For example, for severely traumatized people dissociation may cause the mind to psychologically split into different personality states. This is known as dissociative identity disorder. Within the middle of the dissociation continuum are experiences where you feel emotionally numb and detached and have an altered sense of time, memory lapses, or identity confusion. Depersonalization and derealization are two forms of dissociation.

Depersonalization: You feel a disconnection from your sense of self and your body, as if you're looking at yourself from a distance. You may feel like a robot, cut off from feeling your body's sensations.

Derealization: While depersonalization is the experience of feeling disconnected from yourself and your body, derealization is feeling detached and disconnected from the world around you. You feel as if you're in a dream where things don't seem real.

Do you struggle with any of the above symptoms? If so and they interfere with your life, please consider seeking professional help. These and other C-PTSD symptoms are hard to deal with by yourself, and it's understandable that you've used food to cope. In the "Resources" section, I discuss various trauma-informed therapeutic approaches that can help.

JOURNAL PROMPT

Take a moment and think about the little child you once were. Does anything on this list describe their behavior? You may find it helpful to write your memories in your journal. If reviewing this list is painful, remember to pause, breathe, and perhaps take a walk or do light stretching to move your body. Take a break if necessary. Come back when you're ready.

The above C-PTSD symptoms may be why ending emotional eating has been difficult for you, even when you've been determined to stop. As you're learning, when children experience trauma and abuse—especially chronic abuse—there remains a lack of peace within the body that lasts into adulthood. Physical sensations of fear and stress—the issues in your tissues—may get triggered seemingly out of nowhere. You feel unsettled and unsafe or lose a sense of connection with your body—and yourself—perhaps on a level you don't even notice. You may then emotionally eat and not exactly know why.

A dysregulated nervous system makes it hard to notice your body's deeper needs. Your interoceptive awareness is filled with unsettling trauma-based sensations. Calming your nervous system helps you settle the chaos in your body to better identify your body's needs for certain foods, hydration, rest, sleep, and movement. You're then giving your body what it needs for its health, rather than for your emotional survival.

Learning how to calm your nervous system is key to helping you heal from both early trauma and emotional eating. Thus far you've learned how to breathe diaphragmatically, use progressive muscle relaxation, and visit a peaceful place in your mind. I'll now show you a beautiful self-soothing process I developed to add to your self-care practices.

Give Yourself a Comforting Embrace

In religious and spiritual traditions, the shawl—often used while praying—represents comfort and spiritual shelter. Drawing from this centuries-old tradition, I developed the "Sacred Shawl Practice" to help you calm your body and nervous system and feel grounded in the loving arms of your Wise Self.

Your Wise Self is the part of you that remains unaffected by the trauma you experienced, loves you unconditionally, is ever-present, and is always guiding you to your highest good.

You may think of your Wise Self as your Higher Power, God, Spirit, Consciousness, or Nature. I'll be using the term Wise Self as we proceed with this practice, but use whatever term inspires you.

Sacred Shawl Practice

The following process calls forth your Wise Self to help you feel supported and loved and to lessen fear and worry. You begin to feel protected and safe knowing you're held in the arms of divine love.

Your sacred shawl helps calm your dysregulated body and nervous system. Think of your body as a container. It's holding the trauma-based sensations you experienced in childhood that get triggered today. Self-compassion researcher Kristin Neff (2011), PhD, author of *Self-Compassion: The Proven Power of Being Kind to Yourself*, explains that physical touch and hugs, even when you give them to yourself, can calm stress in the body. Wrapping yourself in your sacred shawl helps reassure your nervous system in the same way a fretful baby feels comforted and secure when swaddled and held in their parent's arms. Here's what you do:

1. Select your shawl.

Look for a beautiful shawl in whatever fabric and pattern you desire. It could be as simple as cotton, as fancy as silk, or a heavier wool. What matters is that you are drawn to it and it's comfortable to wear indoors.

Instead of a shawl, you may prefer to use a shirt, sweater, or even a throw or blanket. I'll refer to shawl, but any garment covering your torso works. Perhaps you already own a special shawl or sweater to use. If not, buy something beautiful just for this purpose.

2. Bless your shawl.

Once you've found the right piece of clothing, you'll now bless it with the divine love of your Wise Self.

Give yourself about thirty minutes of quiet, uninterrupted time in a private space. Sit in a comfortable chair or cross-legged on a cushion if you prefer.

Wrap your sacred shawl around you (or put on whatever garment you're using) and gently wrap your arms around your torso as if to give yourself a hug. Close your eyes (or keep them open if you prefer) and breathe diaphragmatically for a few minutes to calm your mind and settle your body.

Then, say the following prayer silently to yourself or out loud. This prayer invokes the energy and support of your Wise Self. Allow this support to flow through you and your shawl. As you pray, imagine being held in the arms of love.

Dear Wise Self (or Higher Power, God, Spirit),

May this shawl (or shirt, sweater) be blessed with your love and support.

When I feel weak, help me feel strong.

When I feel scared, help me feel grounded.

When I feel worried, help me feel peace.

May I feel safe and secure in the shelter of your loving embrace.

Thank you.

After you say your prayer, sit quietly for a moment. Notice what it's like to feel embraced in your Wise Self's loving presence. Breathe in that energy. Imagine your shawl is infused with this love.

After you bless your sacred shawl with this prayer, you don't need to say it again. Once the loving energy of your Wise Self is invoked, it's always present. But if repeating the prayer deepens your experience, by all means repeat this process. Start with this prayer as a template, but you may choose to use phrases that best resonate with you.

Whenever you put on your sacred shawl, repeat these three affirmations: *I am calm. I am wise. I am peace.*

Saying these affirmations helps you open to receive the loving energy of your Wise Self. You can use these affirmations or choose others that best work for you.

Store your sacred shawl respectfully and keep it visible and readily available to wear. For example, you could lay it on the side of a chair, place it on an open shelf, or keep it in a basket in your bedroom. You may also want to bring it to work or a social event. The beauty of a shawl is that it's a great fashion accessory and no one knows its deeper meaning. For variety and accessibility, you may want to create several sacred shawls so that some can be for private settings and others taken anywhere.

3. Wear your sacred shawl.

Think of your sacred shawl as a spiritual embrace that helps soothe hard feelings, grounds you and calms your nervous system when dysregulated, and also enhances times you already feel settled. Receiving comfort isn't only for stressful times. Much like a child enjoys snuggling with a loving parent simply to feel connected, give yourself regular moments of connection with your Wise Self too.

Here are some suggestions for when to wear your sacred shawl:

- *When you feel triggered to emotionally eat:* Put on your shawl, breathe, and (whether sitting or standing) imagine your loving Wise Self soothing you. Give yourself about ten minutes. To settle yourself further, count your breaths. For example, say to yourself "one," "two," and up to "ten," in synchrony with each out-breath. Repeat as necessary until you feel calmer. Then, decide if you still want to eat. If you do, that's okay and remember to eat mindfully while wearing your shawl for comfort. Remember, this is a process; change takes time. It's not about *not* emotionally eating; it's about how to use self-compassion when you do. (You'll learn more about this in chapter 8.)

- *When stressed and overwhelmed:* Whether or not you're triggered to eat, wear your sacred shawl when you feel worried, sad, or lonely. Sit quietly until you feel settled and soothed. Remember to take gentle diaphragmatic breaths.

- *When you meet with your therapist:* Several of my clients wear their sacred shawl during sessions. It then not only symbolizes support from their Wise Self, but it also becomes associated with growth and healing.

- *While reading this book:* Wearing your sacred shawl can help you feel grounded if triggered.

- *Take it to work:* When feeling stressed, put on your shawl to settle yourself.

- *Deepen moments of self-care:* For example, take a ten-minute break and sip a cup of herbal tea while wearing your shawl. Or wear it while reading a good book, catching up with a close friend on the phone, or listening to music.

Think of your sacred shawl as your spiritual hug. The more you use it, the more ways you'll discover how useful and comforting it feels to wear it. You'll know that helping yourself feel safe and secure is only a hug away.

Putting It All Together

This chapter offered you a foundation to understand how early trauma affected your brain and nervous system. You learned how children react to the fight-flight-freeze-fawn response and how compassionate support, or lack of support, from caretakers affects the child's stress response. You also learned about C-PTSD symptoms and how they contribute to emotional eating. That's a lot of heavy stuff. How are you doing?

I want you to know that despite the challenges of early trauma and C-PTSD, *you can move through this and heal.* With the right tools—including wearing your sacred shawl—you, too, can help your brain and nervous system find peace, which helps you heal emotional eating.

In the next chapter, we'll explore the connection you feel with your body and how to bring love and caring attention to this important relationship. So let's continue.

CHAPTER 4

Connect with Your Body

It's easy to take our bodies for granted or wish they looked different. But when we reflect on everything our body does for us, it's hard not to appreciate the miracle that it is.

Whether able-bodied or with physical challenges, our body gives us many gifts. It can allow us to see, hear, smell, touch, and taste. It allows us to talk and sing, walk and dance, and hold a loved one's hand. Our body allows us to think and make decisions about our life. It is also the container for our emotions, which we experience as physical sensations.

Given the early trauma you experienced, your body has been through a lot. It's important to treat it with compassion for all the pain and trauma it holds.

In previous chapters, you learned about the effects of early trauma on the body. You learned how to calm your body and nervous system by using diaphragmatic breathing, progressive muscle relaxation, and your sacred shawl. These skills and support anchors help you and your body feel grounded and settled, especially when triggered with trauma-based sensations. The more you strengthen your ability to calm your nervous system, the more you build a safe and secure foundation to improve and deepen the relationship you have with your body.

All healthy relationships thrive on mutual respect, loyalty, and trust. Your body needs these relationship-building gifts too. But when you experience the unsettling sensations of a traumatized nervous system, weight cycling from the futility of yo-yo dieting, or harassment from weight stigma, which exacerbates body insecurity, your relationship with your body may suffer.

Take a moment to reflect on your body and answer the following questions. Perhaps you'd like to wear your sacred shawl to feel grounded, get your journal, and write your answers. If focusing on your body feels difficult, that's okay. Just stop, skim through this section, and move on. Do what feels best for you.

- What do you notice is happening in your body right now? Is it calm and settled or uneasy and tense?

- How would you describe your relationship with your body? Is it a relationship filled with love and kindness, or is it fraught with tension? Does your body feel like a best friend or like a stranger or enemy?

- When you think about your body, what feelings emerge? Are they peaceful ones or filled with dislike and shame?

- What beliefs do you hold about your body? Are they beliefs of kindness and acceptance or criticism and self-loathing?

Depending on the relationship you have with your body, these aren't necessarily easy questions. How are you doing? If you need some self-compassion, give yourself a hug with your sacred shawl, breathe, and take a break if necessary.

Body insecurity and emotional eating are often complementary challenges. A history of trauma adds an additional burden because of nervous system dysregulation. Given all of this, it's understandable that you may have a hard time feeling positive about your body.

Body positivity is a popular topic, and I imagine you've read about it. While it holds merit, some people have a hard time believing positive thoughts about their body. I wonder if this applies to you too. If so, that's okay. You feel what you feel. What about trying something different? Instead of forcing yourself to hold a body-positive mindset that doesn't feel true for you, I invite you to practice a *body-supportive* mindset. It may feel easier to think of *supporting your body* rather than trying to feel something you don't feel.

No matter what, you and your body are a team. You are its caretaker, and it relies on you to keep it safe and healthy. You can't feel strong and powerful together if your relationship is fraught with judgment and negativity. Berating yourself and obsessing about your body harms your relationship. To be healthy partners in life, your body needs your support.

It's hard to feel positive about your body if you've been yo-yo dieting and pressuring your body to be something other than what it is. Releasing the grip of expectations to look a certain way or reach a lower weight eases tension you may feel about your body. For example, you begin to pay attention to your *body's* needs rather than *your* need to see a different number on the scale. It means you care more about *your body* than a number that doesn't have anything to do with who you are as a person. In the same way children thrive when feeling accepted for who they are, your body needs your acceptance and support too. Later in this chapter, I'll help you adopt a body-supportive mindset and release the pressure of body expectations.

Let's look at how a body-supportive mindset helped Gloria. Gloria held shame toward her body from the time her brother starting sexually abusing her when she was ten years old. She dissociated during the episodes of abuse and recalled feeling as if she were on the ceiling looking down at herself. This resulted in Gloria feeling detached from her body, and this feeling continued into adulthood. As a higher-weight child, she also was teased, and this exacerbated her feelings of body shame. Food helped her emotionally survive, and she hid sweets in her bureau. After her brother left her bedroom, she turned to cookies to numb her distress.

Given her history, it was impossible for Gloria to hold positive feelings toward her body. "I hated my body," she said. "I blamed it for my brother wanting to touch me. Now I understand that my brother had a problem and what he did had nothing to do with me or my body."

While it took time, and by using the principles in this book, Gloria reclaimed a more nurturing and respectful connection with her body. Even though she felt body shame and insecurity, she became willing to embrace the idea of supporting her body. When Gloria adopted a body-supportive mindset that didn't challenge how she *felt* about her body, she could value the importance of giving her body the care it needed to thrive. This new mindset helped Gloria think about the relationship with her body in a whole new way. Over time, she stopped letting shame and judgment about her body get in the way of caring for it. "After all those years of my body being disrespected," she said, "I'm not going to keep repeating abuse—through my words or actions."

As with Gloria, I want you to understand that *it's not your fault* if it feels impossible to develop a new relationship with your body right now. It's not easy to take care of something you've spent years detaching from, especially when it triggers feelings of shame. And it's hard to feel at peace with a body that creates intense and unpleasant sensations—those "issues in your tissues"—that catch you by surprise.

Offering Your Body Support

When you become willing to support your body, your relationship softens. It moves from a relationship filled with conflict and tension to one of care and respect. You may be critical of your body *and* support its need for tender loving care. It's about expanding your mindset to hold two seemingly opposite thoughts. Notice what it feels like to say the following:

"I may not love my body, *and* I'm willing to take good care of it."

"I'm critical of my body, *and* I can be attentive to its needs."

"I feel ashamed of my body, *and* I can treat it with compassion."

Both sides of each comment can be true, and neither has to negate the other. So please remember this: *you don't have to wait until you love your body before treating it lovingly.*

Write the above statements in your notebook and journal on what it means to adopt a body-supportive mindset, no matter how you feel about your body.

Three Ways to Befriend Your Body

Supporting your body means you're willing to be its friend. You'll now learn three practices to befriend your body and develop the respectful, affectionate connection you both deserve.

1. Connect with Your Body-Wisdom

Your body is always telling you what it needs, even if you don't hear it. As you're learning, dissociation and trauma-based sensations in your body can impede your ability to notice hunger-fullness levels and other signs your body sends about what it needs. The mental chatter of negative thoughts also can block you from hearing your body's guidance. For example, when you're ruminating on self-critical thoughts about your appearance, you're not as open to giving your body the loving attention it needs. Your job is to open lines of communication so you can hear and heed your body's requests.

Your body is more than what you see on the surface. It holds intuitive wisdom that is available when you take time to listen. This wisdom is the same voice as your Wise Self. Connecting with your Wise Self through your body is another pathway to receiving intuitive guidance. When you ask your body-wisdom for guidance, you look beyond the superficial to expand and strengthen your connection with your body.

Your inner wisdom is ever-present. It speaks to you in whispers that you hear not only as thoughts but also as inspired desires. A strong connection with this source of guidance can guide your journey as you improve your relationship with your body and food and heal from child-hood trauma.

Tuning in to your body can feel scary when fear-based sensations of trauma live in your nervous system. That's why it's important to learn how to calm and settle your body through the practices you learned in earlier chapters. As you develop this ability, you also can begin to connect with the guidance of your body-wisdom.

If this is new for you, it may feel strange, or even weird, to think of connecting with your body in this way. That's okay. Just try. Notice what you feel as you read the instructions below. Then practice right now or later when you feel ready. I also made you a recording where I guide you through this process of connecting to your body-wisdom. You can access it here: http://www.newharbinger.com/51178. If practicing now, here's what you do:

1. Start from a place of feeling grounded. Wear your sacred shawl if you wish.

2. Sit in a comfortable chair, in a quiet space, with your back straight and feet firmly on the floor. (After you've practiced and feel comfortable, you may choose to do this while reclin-ing or lying down.)

3. Take a moment to breathe diaphragmatically and settle your-self. Close your eyes or gaze downward.

4. Then, tune in to your body in whatever way feels natural to you. Some people do this by drawing their attention to their heart center or solar plexus.

5. Now, silently to yourself, ask your body the question below. Your body-wisdom communicates to you in whispers. It's a language of silence. You receive information via intuitive nudges, spontaneous insights, or a *feeling* guiding you in a

certain direction. Ask this question in the same way, without noise: *"What do you need from me today so you will feel loved and well-cared for?"*

6. After you ask your body what it needs, stay quiet for a moment. Notice what you hear or sense, if anything. For example, you may hear that your body wants you to rest, drink water, or sign up for that yoga class you've been thinking about. Whatever you hear, do your best to follow through. You may want to get your journal and write about this experience.

When practicing this for the first time, you may not notice a clear message right away. That's not unusual. Connecting with your body like this happens *beyond the mind*, so it may feel as if you have not communicated with it. You may notice a peaceful feeling or subtle whispers of insight emerging later in the day. Or nothing at all. Just know that by being willing to ask and listen to your body's intuitive messages, you open the pathway to receive its guidance. Trust that over time, you'll hear the whispers of your body-wisdom communicating with you. The important thing is to keep asking.

When Gloria first practiced this in a therapy session, she didn't hear a message. But she did feel peaceful. She said, "I didn't *hear* anything but— and this sounds strange—I got the sense that my body was happy I asked the question."

Gloria continued communicating with her body daily. She sometimes heard requests to cook certain foods or go to sleep earlier. She once heard a suggestion to watch her favorite comedy movie for a much-needed break from stress. When Gloria followed through, even when the messages seemed silly, she always felt it was just what she needed.

Emotional safety in any relationship comes from authentic and compassionate communication. Sharing your needs and desires with someone you trust—and you listening to theirs—helps you feel safe with the person and deepens relationships. It's the same with your body. The more you ask what it needs, the more you create a relationship of safety and trust.

Depending on the abuse and trauma you experienced as a child, your body may not have felt loved. You did not feel safe. Asking your body what it needs helps you work together as a trusted team.

When you hear a clear message from your body asking you to do something, it's important to follow through. For example, if you hear a request to drink more water and don't, you are betraying your body by disregarding its request. As in any relationship, honoring your body's wishes keeps your relationship strong.

Once you set your intention to communicate with your body-wisdom on a regular basis, you may notice flashes of insight, subtle urges, or an intuitive feeling nudging you to do something for your body. By taking the time to connect with and listen to your body's messages, these inspiring thoughts and feelings become easier to act on. For example, instead of feeling you "should" exercise after work, you feel inspired to take a walk because you "want" to do something good for your body. When you feel disconnected from your body, you feel obligated to take care of it, but when you feel connected to your body, *you want to take care it.*

As you develop the habit of communicating with your body, over time you'll naturally begin to tune in to your body throughout the day. The loving guidance you receive helps you nurture a more supportive and respectful relationship.

2. Take Your Body for a Walk

I know, you've heard this before. That's because walking is a terrific way to give your body the health benefits of movement. It's also a great way to calm the trauma-based sensations in your body and boost your mood. But I'm not talking about walking for exercise. I want you to think of walking *as a way to make friends with your body.*

Taking your body for a walk is about scheduling quality time with it like you would with a good friend. Think of it as going on a date with your body. Yes, you heard me.

Take your body on a date.

Plan about ten, fifteen, or twenty minutes once a week and take your body for a walk. If walking is hard or you're a person who uses a wheelchair, give your body light stretching or chair-yoga movements.

Whether walking or stretching, do this by yourself. This time is for you and your body and not to be shared with a friend. If possible, walk in a park or by water so you get the added benefits of being in nature. But any place will do.

Since walking calms the nervous system, it can feel easier to focus on your body when you're moving. Walking dates are a good time to get acquainted with your body and develop interoceptive awareness. As you walk, notice what's happening in your body and how it feels. For example, notice how hungry, full, or satisfied you feel. Notice the rhythm of your breathing. Is it rapid and shallow or even and deep? Notice your emotional state. Does your body feel agitated and tense, or peaceful and calm? Draw your attention to your arms and legs as you take each step. Do they feel sluggish and heavy, or sturdy and strong? Notice what's happening in your stomach, back, and head. With a neutral and nonjudgmental mind, simply notice.

Now here's the thing. As you walk, I want you to *talk to your body.* You wouldn't go on a date with a friend and say nothing, would you? Our bodies have a consciousness of their own and respond to our thoughts and words. Talking and sharing builds and deepens relationships. It's the same with your body.

As you walk, here are some things to say (silently or out loud) to your body. When I talk to my body, sometimes I refer to it in the third person, and sometimes I say "us," depending on the situation. Use whatever pronoun works for you.

"Walking is so good for you."

"Our cells thrive on this movement."

"I want to feel connected with you."

"I want you to be happy."

"This is good for us."

Use this time to also offer thanks and appreciation to your body for all it does for you. For example, you can say:

"Thank you, legs for allowing me to walk."

"Thank you, ears for allowing me to hear the birds chirping."

"Thank you, eyes for allowing me to see these beautiful trees."

"Thank you, lungs for breathing."

"Thank you, heart for beating."

Use these and other affirming statements that resonate with you. As you walk, your mind will naturally wander. That's okay. You don't need to say these statements as repetitive mantras. Just stay tuned in to your body as best you can and give it these messages as if you're walking and talking with a friend. And be sure to listen. Notice the whispers of your body-wisdom communicating with you. Maybe you'll hear a message, maybe you won't. Either way, it's okay. Your intention is to spend quality, focused time with your body—with no judgment or expectation—while giving it the gift of connection with movement.

Gloria was skeptical when I suggested that she make a walking date with her body. She normally thought about walking as exercise, so it felt burdensome to her. But she quickly warmed up to the idea. After she had several walking dates with her body, Gloria said, "You know, it was pretty cool. Making a date with my body and talking to it helps me see that it isn't separate from me. I'm in a real relationship with it. I didn't understand what that meant before, but I'm beginning to now."

Weekly walks with your body communicate to both of you that you're making it a priority and want to be its friend. Over time, this helps you honor your body's needs and feel confident about your relationship.

3. Daily Gifts to Your Body

This fun practice boosts your relationship with your body. Simply put, what you do is give your body a daily gift. We all feel loved and appreciated when someone gives us a heartfelt gift for no reason, right? It's the same with your body. Showering it with gifts helps it feel loved.

Daily gifts communicate to your body that it is honored and valued. It doesn't mean you do something extra-special for your body, although you can. The point is to designate one thing each day as your body's gift. For example, your gift can be as luxurious as a hot stone massage, as simple as drinking a glass of water, or an everyday routine, like brushing your teeth. You then mindfully offer caring attention to your body through this gift, even if it's something you do every day. Here are some suggestions of daily gifts for your body:

- Rub lotion on your hands.

- Soak in an aromatherapy bath.

- Soak your feet in Epsom salts.

- Eat a piece of fresh fruit.

- Floss your teeth.

- Listen to a calming meditation.

- Take a nap.

- Breathe deeply for two minutes.

- Dance to your favorite music in your living room.

- Repeat affirmations, such as *"I am healthy, I am strong, I am wise,"* to give your body the gift of uplifting words.

Now let's take this a step further. As you give your body its gift, pair it with a loving statement. For example, while drinking a glass of water, say to your body, "This is so good for you," or when soaking in the tub say, "This soothes your muscles."

The loving intention behind your action is as important as the action itself. Your body absorbs the energy of your thoughts, so instead of merely going through the motions, infuse your actions with nurturing words so you and your body gain the most benefit from your daily gifts.

When you commit to giving your body a daily gift, your mind searches for ways to serve your body better. That's because *we see what we look for.* You begin to naturally scan your environment for things you can do for your body that you may have overlooked before. For example, committing to your daily gift practice may inspire you to park your car farther from the store entrance to give your body the gift of movement or to eat an orange to give your body the gift of vitamin C.

Speaking of movement, the suggestion to park away from a store entrance—certainly a common one—may send off alarm bells if you're feeling diet-weary and cringe at anything that feels like pressure to exercise. If you can relate, would you be willing to think about movement differently? Our thoughts are powerful and guide our actions, so even a slight shift in thinking can make a big difference. Since moving your body helps your body—and is vital for its well-being—it's important to not let old triggers stop you from giving your body the movement it deserves. Begin to release the heavy associations you may hold with the word "exercise" so your body receives the benefits of movement. How about thinking of movement as a *loving gift* to your body? Your body will thank you, and you will appreciate the invigorating results that movement gives you. (Unless they got injured, no one ever said, "I regret taking that walk.")

When I suggested the daily gift practice to Gloria, she loved the idea and committed to giving her body a month of daily gifts. She told her best friend about it, and they did it together. They shared gift ideas and texted each other daily after giving their body its gift. Perhaps you would like to share this idea with a friend too. It helps you both stay accountable and adds to the fun.

Unless you're inspired to begin with one month as Gloria did, I suggest you start small with one week of daily gifts. Maybe you'll decide to jump right in today or wait until you finish this book. Whenever you begin, use a journal to record your daily gifts and write down what it feels like to give this gift to your body. Recording your gifts helps you see progress and stay committed. (You can download the "Daily Gifts to My Body" checklist at http://www.newharbinger.com/51178.)

Giving your body a daily gift is a fun and beautiful way to shower it with kindness. Instead of battling with your body, you become best friends.

A Supportive Relationship with Your Body

Along with the grounding and self-compassion practices you learned in earlier chapters, in this chapter you learned three ways to connect with your body to nurture a respectful partnership. As you commit to taking these steps, over time you'll begin to relate to your body in a more compassionate and supportive way.

To help you gauge your progress, below are five signs you're creating a more supportive relationship with your body. After reading each one, ask yourself the follow-up question to note the quality of connection you have with your body today. Each question asks for self-rating on a one-to-ten scale, with an example at both ends. Answer as best you can and record your answer. You may want to date and write this in your journal monthly to monitor progress.

1. You and your body can relax.

Adult survivors of trauma often find it difficult to let their guard down, even in peaceful situations. It's hard to feel a positive connection with your body—and listen to its intuitive messages—when you and your body are always on edge.

You'll know you're feeling a safer connection with your body as you experience moments of relaxation and calm, unaided by food.

On a scale of one to ten, with one being very relaxed and ten being highly tense, how do you rate the level of relaxation or tension you feel in your body right now? Based on your answer, what, if any, action will you take? (For example, if you feel tense you can take five diaphragmatic breaths.)

2. You notice–and heed–your body's sensations of hunger, fullness, and thirst.

When you feel disconnected from your body, you're less apt to recognize and attend to your body's need for food and hydration.

You'll know you're feeling a supportive connection with your body as you hold a clearer awareness of your body's internal signals. You'll not only notice how your body feels when it's hungry and full, you'll honor what it needs and give it the right amount of nourishment.

Using the hunger-fullness scale (in chapter 2), notice how hungry or full you feel right now. Additionally, on a scale of one to ten, with one being "I'm not thirsty" and ten being "I'm very thirsty," how do rate your body's hydration need? Based on your answers, what action, if any, will you take?

3. You hear your body-wisdom.

Subtle sensations are one way your body-wisdom speaks to you. Your body is the portal through which you notice a gut feeling, inner warning sign, or sense of truth about a situation. Your intuition often speaks to you quietly, in whispers. Anxiety and trauma-based sensations in your body can block you from receiving these messages. They're always there. It's just harder to notice them. But you can strengthen your inner guidance receptors by intentionally connecting with your body-wisdom as you learned above.

You'll know you're developing a supportive and safe connection with your body as you begin to notice your intuition speaking to you. You'll sense and feel this in your body, mind, and spirit as a subtle inner knowing.

As you heed your inner guidance—which always wants to support you—it gently leads you forward along your healing journey.

On a scale of one to ten, with one being completely unaware and ten being highly aware, how do you rate your ability to hear your intuition communicating with you? Based on your answer, what, if any, action will you take? (For example, if it's hard to hear your intuition, practice the body-wisdom exercise.)

4. You notice signs your body needs care, and you take action.

It's hard to take care of a body you feel detached from. This affects *all* your self-care and hygiene decisions, not only your food choices. For example, you may be lax about flossing your teeth or showering, or feel you don't deserve to use the luxurious hand lotion you got for your birthday.

Your body lets you know what it needs. Your job is to notice. When you feel a supportive connection with your body, you're aware of physical changes before they turn serious, feeling tired before you're exhausted, and that you need to de-stress before your clenched jaw causes a migraine. You take action as necessary.

A supportive connection with your body means you follow through with whatever routine preventive health care is available to you, such as annual physicals, dental cleanings, and appropriate screenings. It also means you pamper yourself in small yet meaningful ways. For example, using that hand lotion, giving yourself a manicure, or soaking your sore feet in Epsom salts.

On a scale of one to ten, with one being "I neglect my body's needs" and ten being "I take excellent care of my body's needs," how do you rate the level of care you give your body? Based on your answer, what action, if any, will you take?

5. You allow stressful emotions to flow through your body.

Given your history of childhood trauma, it's understandable that you may have a hard time tolerating your feelings. When intense emotion strikes and your body reacts, it can bring you right back to feeling like a vulnerable, scared child. Your impulse has been to numb the emotion with food.

When you feel a safe connection with your body, you'll feel less afraid of intense emotion and trust your ability to cope. Instead of impulsively turning to food—although you still may at times—you use other ways to soothe your feelings.

On a scale of one to ten, with one being "I cannot tolerate any hard feeling" and ten being "I am able to embrace and be with *all* of my feelings," how do you rate your ability to welcome and be present with your feelings? (Don't worry if this feels hard for you right now. You'll learn how to mindfully process feelings in chapter 6.)

Putting It All Together

This chapter focused on your body, and that can feel hard when you hold painful or confusing feelings about it. How are you doing? Perhaps you'd like to take a break and write in your journal about what has come up for you.

You learned three practices—connecting with your body-wisdom, taking your body for a walk, and giving it a daily gift—all designed to help you develop a respectful partnership and relate with your body as the sacred partner it's meant to be. Have fun with these! If you feel inspired, practice all three at the same time. Or start with one. Perhaps you'd like to begin by thinking about a gift to give your body today. Or maybe you could get quiet and ask your body what it needs from you right now. Or take your body on a five-minute walking date today. Keep it simple and consistent.

Every few months, revisit the five signs to gauge how your relationship with your body is progressing. Remember, creating a strong connection with your body is a *practice*. And developing new practices, which you're learning in this book, takes time, patience, and perseverance. Above all else, be gentle with yourself. Hold faith in your heart.

You'll get there.

Thus far, we've discussed how trauma has affected your physical body. In the next chapter, we'll explore the unseen yet powerful world of trauma-based beliefs, which can trigger emotional eating, and how to release these beliefs so they no longer hold you back from living the life you deserve. So let's continue.

CHAPTER 5

Cultivate Inner Emotional Safety

To accomplish anything in your life—including healing emotional eating—you must first expect it for yourself *and feel safe to receive it.* I'm not referring to your physical safety, although that's essential. I'm talking about feeling *emotionally safe.* It's hard to create change unless you believe that you're worthy to accept the changes you want to make. Disempowering beliefs that sabotage your self-worth—conscious or subconscious—are sneaky. They hold you back without you even knowing. But once you identify and transform them, they'll lose their power, and you'll be on your way.

When we begin to transition from familiar ways of coping, we may feel resistance. It's as if you're at a border crossing and don't know what's on the other side. Fear and self-doubt yell at you to turn around. But when you feel emotionally safe inside, you not only feel inspired to create new habits, but *you expect to succeed*—no matter how loudly fears yell.

Let's look at how your conscious and subconscious minds can work together so you feel safe to cross that border and heal emotional eating and childhood trauma.

Your conscious mind guides many of your choices, but it's your subconscious mind that influences the outcome of everything. How you feel about yourself deep inside affects every aspect of your life, including healing emotional eating, self-care, building relationships, and even managing your money. That's because your subconscious mind is much more powerful than your conscious mind.

Think of your subconscious as a container that holds the messages you received and feelings you experienced when you were a child. When children are treated with love, respect, and kindness, they are more likely to feel valuable and worthy. Feelings and beliefs of positive self-regard are deposited into their container and held for a lifetime. These inner resources are available to draw from when needed. If you didn't get these positive resources early on, that's okay because *it's never too late to change that*. This chapter teaches you a process to help you create inner emotional safety even if you didn't experience it earlier in life.

Children from functional and loving families are challenged by life's trials like everyone, but deep inside they rely on their foundation of positive self-worth. All children, whether traumatized or not, hold some limiting beliefs. That's being human. But when children feel emotionally and physically safe growing up, they head into adulthood with their conscious and subconscious minds mostly aligned, which helps them live a fulfilling life despite challenges and stress.

When children and teens are traumatized, however, particularly when the trauma is abuse or neglect, their world isn't safe. Powerless to stop what's happening, they may feel fear and helplessness—often daily. Burying these feelings helps them survive. The psychological defense mechanisms that push feelings away are called suppression and repression. Suppression is when you consciously avoid thoughts and feelings that are too hard to deal with. It's like putting dirty laundry in a drawer. You know it's there but don't think about it.

Repression is an unconscious process where the mind blocks the awareness of difficult thoughts and feelings and deposits, or represses, them into the subconscious and out of awareness of the conscious mind. It's like burying the dirty laundry and forgetting it ever existed. Suppression and repression of fear-based feelings (along with dissociation that you learned about in chapter 3) are necessary defense mechanisms. They helped you survive.

On the surface, some traumatized children may seem okay (although others reveal chronic sadness on their faces), while inside they carry fear and pain. Abused and neglected children begin to believe that they are unworthy of love and protection. Their subconscious mind—their inner container—fills with beliefs of low self-worth and fear, and as you learned in earlier chapters, their body holds these emotions as disquieting physical sensations that easily can be triggered.

When children feel safe to tell a trusted adult that they're being harmed and are then protected, or have someone to talk with about a death, divorce, or other family crisis, they no longer bear the burden of burying their feelings. With support from family members and perhaps professionals, they are free to talk. Even if talking feels hard at first, they know that *they are seen*. Receiving support and validation helps them feel loved. The shame and fear held in their subconscious container then can be replaced, or at least counterbalanced, with feelings of positive self-worth and emotional safety.

If you didn't have anyone to help you or talk to when you were a child, your subconscious mind emotionally protected you. When it wasn't safe to express your fear and despair, these feelings took shelter and hid in your subconscious. It would have been even *more* painful and scary to acknowledge the enormity of these feelings when you were little and alone, so your mind cleverly put these feelings in your container—out of view from your conscious mind—to help you get through the day. For example, when a child knows that they may be lashed with a belt by Mom or Dad at any moment, they can't focus on that daily without making themselves sick. The fear of what's possible goes underground so they can emotionally survive.

This doesn't mean you didn't feel *any* of that pain or fear. I'm sure you did. Most likely, the protection your subconscious mind gave you just made that unbearable pain easier to bear.

These painful feelings expand into beliefs and hide in the child's subconscious container as they move into adulthood. Because of this, their conscious and subconscious minds do not always align. Instead, they often compete with one another.

But the desires of the conscious mind are no match for the might of the subconscious mind. Hidden beneath the surface, your subconscious holds *all* your emotional memories—in your mind and in your body—making it much more powerful than your conscious mind.

Think of it this way: The captain of the ship (you) wants to go in a certain direction (stop relying on food to cope). But no matter how forcefully the captain shouts orders, unless the crew (your subconscious fears and beliefs) complies with the captain's plan, the boat (your actions) will go where the crew wants to go. The conflict sounds something like this:

Conscious mind: "I want to stop using food to cope."

Subconscious mind: "No way. I need food to cope."

Your subconscious container is filled with a crew of fears, blocking you from reaching your destination. These fears include any trauma-based feeling or limiting belief that triggers emotional eating or stops you from living your best life. You may be aware of some fears yet unaware of others. To discover hidden beliefs, examine your behavior. For example, Damian prided himself as a man who "goes with the flow." After self-reflection and learning about the fawn stress response, he realized that being overly flexible protected him from disappointing people and risking their rejection. He hadn't connected his eating habits with the stress created by dishonoring his needs. He thought he just liked to eat.

As you read this book, your awareness may expand to help you dig deeper and uncover hidden fears. For now, just focus on the ones that are obvious to you. Either known or hidden, in response to your desire to heal emotional eating, these fears mutiny with disempowering thoughts to stop you. But you can stop *them* by changing these thoughts into empowering ones.

Changing, or reframing, your thoughts is a cognitive behavioral therapy (CBT) technique. Psychiatrist Aaron Beck developed CBT in the 1960s and discovered how reframing our thoughts improves our mood and supports behavior change. Simply put, reframing means you consciously change a limiting belief to one that feels hopeful and uplifting. Repeating this new, reframed thought retrains your brain to think in less limiting and more positive ways. The more you repeat it, the more open you become to believing it. When I help clients reframe their thoughts, I suggest new ones that are a slight stretch but feel within reach. For example, if you believe, *I'll never stop emotionally eating*, it's unrealistic to reframe that thought to *I no longer emotionally eat*. That's too big a jump. But thinking, *It will take time, but with patience and perseverance I can heal emotional eating*, feels possible to achieve, doesn't it? It still may feel like a stretch for some, but chances are, this reframe offers the promise of success. This is how reframing limiting thoughts and beliefs helps you create new ways of behaving. When your mind moves from despair to inner trust, you're more likely to take positive, self-affirming actions.

While CBT is a helpful strategy, reframing trauma-based thoughts via cognition alone is not necessarily enough. That's why I created the sacred vessel practice below. For new thoughts to take root and grow, you need to water them with love.

Let's first delve deeper and get to know your crew of fears better. Below are ten common disempowering beliefs and fears that traumatized people who use food to cope often struggle with. These thoughts can trigger binge-eating episodes, undermine your relationship with food and your body, and erode your self-worth. But once you become acquainted with them, they'll begin to lose their power and you'll regain yours.

On the left side of the box are fear-based beliefs and related feelings. On the right are new, reframed thoughts to soften these fears. While you may not relate to all of them, some may feel familiar.

Fear-Based Beliefs and Feelings	Reframed Thoughts
I won't stop using food to cope. It's too scary. (Fear, anxiety.)	I don't have to stop completely. To feel safe, I can adjust slowly.
I hate my body. (Self-loathing, shame.)	It's okay to feel how I feel about my body. I don't have to love my body to give it support and kindness.
People hurt you. (Hypervigilance, loneliness, emotional isolation.)	Just because some people in my life hurt me, doesn't mean everyone will. And even if someone does, I'll be okay.
I'm unlovable. (Shame, self-loathing.)	I was not treated lovingly, but that doesn't mean I'm unlovable. I can learn to give myself the love I deserve.
I'm afraid I can't stop emotionally eating. I've tried so many times and failed. (Shame, hopelessness.)	Each new day gives me the chance to make new choices.
I'm afraid of disappointing people. (Fear, hypervigilance.)	It's okay to do what's best for me. Other people's feelings are not my responsibility.
It takes too much effort to care for my body. (Helplessness.)	I deserve to put time and energy into taking care of myself. As I do, it will feel easier.
I don't deserve to be happy. (Low self-worth.)	We all deserve to be happy— including me.
Change is too hard. (Helplessness, hopelessness.)	Sure, change can feel hard. And I'm worth the effort.
Food is the only thing that brings me comfort. (Hopelessness.)	Food gives me comfort, and other things give me comfort too.

What was it like to read this list? Can you identify with some of these limiting beliefs? If so, I want to reassure you that you're not alone. These fears and beliefs are common for people who were traumatized as children and struggle with emotional eating. If you feel triggered, give yourself a dose of self-compassion: pause, breathe, and hug yourself with your sacred shawl.

If other disempowering beliefs come to mind, write them in your journal. Be sure to also write a softer reframe next to each one. If it's hard to create reframes on your own, use this general affirming statement for each limiting belief you identify: "Even though I've carried this inside for a long time, it doesn't mean it's true. I can learn to think differently now."

Perhaps you're thinking, *But the abuse (or neglect or trauma) happened so long ago. How can it still affect me today?* As far as your subconscious mind is concerned, the amount of time that has passed doesn't matter. In the same way your body is like a time capsule holding the physical sensations of trauma, your subconscious mind holds the beliefs you internalized when you were living through that turmoil. These disempowering beliefs remain inside you until they're safely processed and released. That's why when you're triggered, your reactions can feel as intense today as they did years ago.

Let's look at how Clarissa's trauma history affected her beliefs, feelings, and relationship with food. Clarissa entered therapy after the man she dated for one year ended their relationship. Using food was her main way to cope, so emotional eating episodes increased. Clarissa was experiencing panic, grief, and feelings of abandonment. Food helped numb her feelings as she questioned why yet another relationship ended.

While Clarissa enjoyed professional success and close friendships, her relationship history revealed short-lived connections. Her parents separated when she was nine years old. Even when parents are sensitive to their children's needs, a family breakup is still traumatizing for children. (An exception may be when a child or teenager is relieved that their parents' separation means a peaceful or nonviolent life.) In Clarissa's situation, it wasn't only that the separation was traumatic. It was that no one talked about it.

Clarissa learned one Friday evening that her father had moved out. When he didn't return from work, she asked where he was. Her mother said he was living with Grandpa and that she would see him next weekend. Clarissa learned not to question her mother—the family "no talk" rule was clear—but she defied the rule and asked, "What do you mean he's living with Grandpa?" Her mother said, "I told you. Your father isn't living here anymore. Now do your homework."

At school on Monday, Clarissa didn't say anything to her classmates or teachers. She stopped inviting friends over because she didn't know how to explain where her father was. And she had a disturbing feeling that her mother had a boyfriend.

Clarissa lived with these two secrets for four years—that her father wasn't home and her mother was having an affair—pretending to friends and extended family that nothing changed. She saw her father on weekends but never discussed with him what was happening. It took emotional energy to hide her confusion and sadness. She felt worthless and thought, *Dad left because he doesn't love me anymore.* She felt worried and thought, *I hope Cousin Virginia doesn't ask about Dad at Thanksgiving.* She felt guilty and thought, *Dad doesn't know I know that Mom has a boyfriend.* For years, Clarissa and her family acted as if nothing changed. Cookies and candy soothed her sadness.

When Clarissa was thirteen and her parents' divorce finalized, she learned her instinct was true. Returning home from school, she found a strange man watching television in the living room. Her mother said, "This is Jack." No more was said. Clarissa recalls Jack entering her mother's bedroom that night and how sick she got from eating too many peanut butter cups.

Even if Clarissa had been able to discuss the separation and divorce with her parents, she still would have felt the trauma of her family breakup. But not talking about it and living a secretive life added another layer of trauma. Whether the trauma is abuse, neglect, family alcoholism, divorce, or death, not talking about it creates profound inner turmoil. Children and teens can move through many childhood traumas if they have adult support. But trauma, coupled with not talking about that trauma, adds another layer of emotional mayhem.

Consequently, as an adult Clarissa struggled with many disempowering beliefs, including these:

- People you love leave you.

- My feelings don't matter.

- I'm not worthy of love.

- You can't trust people.

- I can't depend on anyone. I must take care of myself.

Early trauma can affect all parts of someone's life or specific aspects. While Clarissa enjoyed a fulfilling career and close friendships, the main area of turmoil was in her intimate relationships. Her subconscious fear of abandonment and rejection, coupled with her belief that it wasn't safe to depend on others, led her to choose emotionally unavailable partners and avoid relationships for long periods of time. These fears never meant to hurt her; they were only trying to keep her safe. The underlying belief was *If you don't connect, you don't get hurt.*

Using food to self-soothe helped Clarissa ease feelings of unworthiness, abandonment, and rejection that often were triggered while dating someone and intensified after the relationship ended. As she learned about the effects of childhood trauma, Clarissa began to understand why she was hypersensitive to rejection and abandonment and why, in those moments, she felt like that little girl who longed for her daddy.

Befriending Your Fears

In the same way Clarissa's fears ruled her life, it's your subconscious fears and limiting beliefs that—for now—hold power over you. But once they're revealed and you understand how they get in your way, you can begin to take charge of them. Understanding isn't only a mental process. It's an emotional one too. As you learn how to *love and soothe* these fears rather than push them away with food, they'll cease to control your life.

One way to take charge of these fears is to look at them with new eyes. What if your fears don't want to frighten you, but want to protect you? What if they're trying to help you feel a sense of control over situations in which you once felt helpless?

Think of it this way: Fear-based beliefs enter your life wanting to be your friends. They often emerge as a signal for safety. For example, you fear getting hit by a car, so you don't run across a highway. You fear getting burned, so you don't put your hand on a hot stove. But fears and beliefs aren't only about the obvious. They develop from our early relationships. Clarissa felt abandoned by her father and betrayed by her mother. Her subconscious mind didn't want her to feel that way again, so it built a wall of fear-based beliefs around her heart to keep her safe. This kept Clarissa as emotionally unavailable as the men she met. And food eased her fear. There was nothing "wrong" with Clarissa eating yummy brownies when she felt lonely and rejected. The problem was that, as you learned earlier, relying on food alone kept her from healing the underlying pain.

Like Clarissa, your fears—both conscious and subconscious—grew out of a need to survive. When a child is abused and her world is a scary place, she's smart to fear the world. When a child learns that nothing she says or does prevents her mother from drinking, her father from leaving, or her coach from criticizing her body, she's smart to fear and distrust the adults in her life. When a child learns that food—not people—can be trusted to soothe her feelings and calm her anxious body, she's smart to seek food when distressed. That's resourceful, not weak-minded.

So I want you to remember this: You're not a vulnerable little child anymore. You have resources now that you didn't have when you were a child. *You no longer need to feel afraid.*

Whether you experienced trauma as a child or adult, the idea of losing food as your comforting friend may trigger unsettling emotions. Instead of feeling optimistic as you make positive changes, you may feel the opposite. For example, you may experience a sense of loss or grief about letting go of old habits. As you begin to relate to food more mindfully, you may feel sadness or anxiety that your relationship with "your friends" is changing. If you begin to feel this way, understand that it's normal and shows that you're healing. Even when someone who has been chronically depressed starts to feel better, they may feel sadness about letting go of depression. It's like giving up an old, comfortable coat. I know this sounds counterintuitive, but a sense of loss or fear is not unusual when you're healing and changing. It's hard to let go of the familiar even when the familiar has been painful.

I want you to know that difficult feelings—your crew of fears—will challenge you as you release your need to use food for comfort. *That's okay.* You're still the captain of your ship. When food has felt like your best friend, it's normal to fear changing that relationship. Change *is* unsettling. But remember, underneath these fears is a wellspring of strength and courage too.

Soothing Your Fears

To release your subconscious crew of fears and limiting beliefs, you need to "hold" them with tenderness, just as you would hold and comfort a child who feels scared and alone. Fears gain strength when you try to push them away. You can't release them permanently without *soothing them first.*

How do you soothe them without food? With love. I developed the following mindful self-compassion practice to help you do this.

Create Your Sacred Vessel

As you've learned, your subconscious is like an inner container carrying the fear-based beliefs you experienced when you were a child. You had no choice because that's how children develop. They're emotional sponges absorbing the words spoken and emotional climate around them. But you have choices today that you didn't have then and can now change these beliefs. To help you heal these hidden stirrings, I'd like you to *bring your subconscious into physical form* and find a real container—your sacred vessel—to symbolize your inner one.

This exercise creates a spiritual healing pathway to your subconscious. You're sending love, compassion, and mindful presence to fear, disempowering beliefs, and self-judgment. Practicing healing rituals with sincere intention helps you develop confidence and inner trust because you're harnessing not only your thoughts but *your heart*. Rituals also help boost self-worth and calm your nervous system because you're setting aside quiet, reflective time to care for yourself. My clients report feeling a sense of peace, hopefulness, and empowerment when they practice their sacred vessel ritual. I think you will too.

Step 1. Find a Special Container

For your sacred vessel, choose a container with a lid to keep the contents protected. (If you can't find one with a lid, that's okay. You can drape a piece of pretty fabric over the top.) You'll be filling your container with pieces of paper and small objects, so be sure it has a fairly wide opening. For example, your sacred vessel could be a patterned cardboard box or woven basket.

To keep your sacred vessel's energy pure, consider buying a new container. But if you own something you'd like to use because it holds meaning for you, that's fine. Just be sure that the memories associated with it are positive or neutral.

Think of this container as a holy vessel that holds your precious inner world—and the inner world you experienced when you were a child. While you carry these thoughts and beliefs within your mind, heart, and body, this external symbol helps create some emotional distance from them. You also may want to put a photo of yourself when you were a child or teenager next to your sacred vessel. That way, you're holding your inner child in your consciousness during your practice.

Put your sacred vessel in a safe and easily accessible spot in your home. If you live with others, ask them to not handle or misuse it.

Step 2. Honor Your Crew of Fears

Once you find your sacred vessel, it's time to name your crew of fears. Remember, you're the captain of your ship. Your fears don't want to hurt you. They simply want your reassurance and love. While they once were there to help you, remind yourself that you no longer need that kind of help anymore.

Give yourself about one hour of uninterrupted time for this step. You may want to wear your sacred shawl or light a candle to create a sense of nurturing comfort. It's possible that you may feel triggered by identifying your crew of fears. That's okay. You don't need to fear being triggered. You just need to know how to comfort yourself when you are. Remember to use diaphragmatic breathing and give yourself a firm, warm hug with your sacred shawl if you feel anxious. This may not happen, but you'll be prepared just in case.

Here's what you do:

1. Get a few sheets of plain paper. Cut them into strips about one- or two-inches wide and four- to five-inches long. You'll be writing each fear-based belief on one strip. Keep one uncut piece of paper to list the achievable reframes.

2. On each strip of paper—one by one—write the fears and limiting beliefs that you hold. Use the ones listed above or any others unique to you. After writing each limiting belief, and before moving to the next one, take the uncut piece of paper and write its corresponding reframed thought. For example, after

writing on one strip of paper, "I'm afraid I can't stop emotionally eating. I've tried so many times and failed," take the uncut paper and write, "Each new day gives me the chance to make new choices." After writing the reframe, repeat it to yourself to set the intention of where you're headed. Continue that way for each limiting belief and its new reframe.

3. If you add limiting beliefs not on the above list, do your best to create a new reframe that feels authentic. If you have difficulty doing that, use this general one I suggested above, which for many people feels achievable: "Even though I've carried this inside for a long time, it doesn't mean it's true. I can learn to think and feel differently now."

4. Set aside the piece of paper with the reframed thoughts for later.

5. Once you've written your crew of fears on individual strips of paper, add them to your sacred vessel, one by one. After you've added them, close the lid, and put your hands on or around your sacred vessel and repeat the following affirming statement three times. *"I am not these fears, and these fears are not me. They're just thoughts and feelings I carry inside, and they need my love."*

6. Then, say the following prayer—silently to yourself or out loud—while imagining the golden light of love from your Wise Self flowing into your container and embracing your fears and disempowering beliefs:

Dear Wise Self, please hold these fears and thoughts in your loving embrace. Thank you.

7. Stay quiet for a moment while holding your sacred vessel. Breathe. Notice how being present with these thoughts and beliefs takes away some of their power. Then, put down your sacred vessel. Trust that you've now enlisted spiritual and loving energies to help you cultivate inner emotional safety.

(To make them easy to remember, you may want to write down the affirming statement and prayer on a small card and keep it near your sacred vessel.)

Step 3. Choose Your Love Energy

In this step, you'll add love to your sacred vessel whenever your crew of fears cries out. To do this, choose items or materials that feel like healing energy to you.

For example, you can use ribbon or small strips of pretty fabric, glass beads, or small stones or shells. Or, simply write the word "love" on small pieces of paper. Clarissa used six-inch strips of different colored ribbons. They reminded her of her devoted grandmother who used ribbons to braid her hair.

Put whatever love materials you use in a special box or bag placed next to your sacred vessel. You'll want them available for when your crew of fears needs your attention.

Take the paper with the reframed thoughts and place it under or near the love materials so it's readily available to review as needed.

Step 4. Soothe Your Fears with Love

Once you find the materials for your love energy, activate your sacred vessel by giving love to your crew of fears.

Place one ribbon, stone, or the word "love" written on paper—whatever love material you decide to use—into your sacred vessel.

Then cradle your hands around your sacred vessel while repeating the prayer from step 2. Again, imagine the golden light of your Wise Self flowing into your container and holding your fears with love and tenderness as you say silently to yourself or out loud:

Dear Wise Self, please hold these fears and thoughts in your loving embrace. Thank you.

Sit quietly for a moment. Breathe.

Then, as you again cradle your sacred vessel in your hands, repeat the following affirmation from step 2 three times to set in motion the healing power of love: *"I am not these fears, and these fears are not me. They're just thoughts and feelings I carry inside, and they need my love."*

Breathe.

Step 5. Keep Adding Love

When you feel gripped by fear-based, disempowering thoughts, and especially when triggered to emotionally eat, practice step 4 and add love and healing energy to your sacred vessel. You may find that this simple act of mindful self-compassion softens or eliminates the urge to eat and helps you better deal with what triggered you. If you decide to eat afterward though, that's okay. This won't necessarily stop you from emotionally eating, although it may. Mostly, it's about being mindfully present with hard thoughts and beliefs and embracing them—and yourself—with love. If you're away from home when triggered, add love when you return.

You don't need to add love only to counterbalance fear. Use your sacred vessel daily or weekly. There are no boundaries to giving your inner world love and self-compassion. So give generously.

Step 6. Continue the Practice

As you move along your healing journey, keep reframing your beliefs to align with the person you're becoming and make corresponding changes with your sacred vessel. For example, Clarissa noticed that she was not as triggered by feelings of rejection. While she felt "unlovable" at times, the feeling was less intense. This correlated with fewer binge-eating episodes. To complement her emotional progress, I suggested that Clarissa remove from her sacred vessel the strip of paper with "I'm not worthy of love" written on it and write it again but on a smaller strip. Clarissa added this new, smaller one back to her sacred vessel and discarded the original.

Making the strip smaller helped Clarissa affirm that she was healing. Each time she became aware of a fear or limiting belief softening, she did the same thing. Ultimately, the strips of paper in her sacred vessel—her crew of fears—became smaller and smaller. And love got bigger and bigger.

Make similar adjustments to your sacred vessel to acknowledge when fears or limiting beliefs no longer hold the same power over you. Congratulate yourself and remember to thank your Wise Self for helping you heal your fears with love.

To develop awareness of the inner shifts you're making, occasionally—perhaps monthly—ask yourself the following questions:

- What fears feel less intense?

- What limiting beliefs feel less powerful?

- In what ways am I feeling more confident?

Pay attention to how often you add love to your sacred vessel and what that feels like. Notice the moment when you realize that there's less fear and more love. If your sacred vessel fills up, feel free to find a larger one so you can keep adding more love.

Putting It All Together

This chapter helped you identify trauma-based beliefs and fears that trigger emotional eating and create roadblocks to healing. You learned how to make and use a sacred vessel to cultivate inner emotional safety and love the parts of you that have felt scared and hurt for so long.

I want you to know that developing inner strength, confidence, and self-trust isn't about *not* feeling fear. It's about learning how to feel strong, confident, and trusting *with* fear. So have faith. Fear-based beliefs don't need to be released quickly or entirely for you to take charge of them. The sacred vessel ritual helps you stay present *with* these fears and beliefs while offering them love and support to loosen their hold over you.

Now that you learned how to befriend limiting beliefs so they no longer hijack your healing, in the next chapter, you'll learn how to mindfully process your feelings, especially feelings rooted in early trauma and trigger the urge to eat.

CHAPTER 6

Process Your Feelings Mindfully

Our feelings make us human. They allow us to experience a rich life. While some feelings are hard to be with, others are light and easy. Either way, feelings simply *are*. They're neither good nor bad. What matters is how you relate to your feelings. You've probably gotten very good at distancing yourself from some, while other feelings overwhelm you. For example, you may push away sadness and grief yet often experience worry and fear. Some feelings may trigger overreactions, especially when your body becomes dysregulated, for example, when minor annoyances trigger a rush of adrenaline and you lash out in anger. Early trauma can wreak havoc on your ability to process feelings in a healthy way. But the good news is that learning about your feelings is like learning a new language, and it's never too late to do that.

Knowing and owning your feelings make you an emotionally whole and aware human being. When you're disconnected from your feelings, you're disconnected from *yourself*. But when you're connected with your feelings, you're more in charge of yourself and, therefore, your life. When you allow yourself to accept and feel *all* of your feelings, you can trust yourself. You then take better care of yourself because you know what you need.

Your feelings are the pathway to healing. Think of them as your guides. Ask yourself right now, "What am I feeling?" Are you feeling happy, sad, angry? Feelings produce a physical response, so tune in to your body too. What sensations do you notice? Are you aware of any tension or tightness, or relaxation and calm? Just notice. If you don't know what you're feeling, that's okay. Simply asking helps you better know yourself. As you learn to welcome all of your feelings—and as hard as it may seem at first—your emotional-eating-healing and trauma-healing journey becomes easier.

Let's start learning the language of feelings by understanding the difference between emotions, feelings, and states.

Although often used interchangeably (as I do for simplicity's sake), there is a difference between an emotion and a feeling. As you've learned, the body produces physiological sensations associated with our thoughts and beliefs. These sensations can be described as emotion. For example, a sinking feeling in your gut, trembling hands, or lightness of spirit.

Your mind interprets and names the emotion in your body as a feeling. Everyone's interpretation is unique to their circumstances. For example, you name the sinking feeling "sadness" because you quarreled with your friend, trembling hands as "fear" because you're awaiting concerning test results, and lightness of spirit as "joy" because you're watching your child play.

Think of it this way: emotion is a physical message in your body, and feeling is what you name it.

Sometimes we feel things that we can't associate with a situation. We're less confused when these are uplifting feelings. For example, when you feel happy "for no reason," you normally don't question that. But harder feelings without a "reason" may seem confusing. This often relates to anxiety or depression. While often called feelings, when anxiety and depression are persistent, they're described as "states."

Chronic moderate to severe depression is a state of numbness or frozen feeling. It's often the embodiment of unprocessed and unreleased pain—sadness, grief, despair—that is held within the body, mind, and nervous system. Depending on the level of severity, one way to relieve depression is by "thawing out" these frozen feelings and *feeling* them. When someone has experienced early trauma with no ability to process pain, they may live in a state of depression that is so familiar they don't realize they're depressed.

Anxiety is also considered a "state" when it is persistent and there is no situational trigger. For example, you may fear flying, so you're anxious about an upcoming trip. The anxiety ends once you safely land. A state of anxiety, however, can emerge for no obvious reason and persist. Sometimes anxiety is a "signal" of unprocessed feelings coming to the surface. Once the deeper feelings emerge and are processed, anxiety may lift.

When depression and anxiety are severe and persist, however, and therapeutic approaches don't offer relief, medication therapy (or higher levels of care) may be necessary. It's unfortunate that there is still stigma around this. If medication has been suggested to you for anxiety or depression and you feel uncomfortable taking it, I hope you will reconsider and explore its benefits with your health care provider.

Now that you know the difference between emotions, feelings, and states, let's look at some common feelings traumatized children experience. Some children have adult support to acknowledge their feelings, receive comfort, and talk about their pain and fears. This is what it means to process feelings so they can be released. But many traumatized children do not have this help. When unprocessed, trauma-based feelings remain inside the child's mind, body, and nervous system into adulthood. Even when a child has help to process their feelings, some traumatic feelings may remain. As you read the following list, notice the feelings that you may persistently experience today. Chances are that some, if not all, of these feelings prompt your urge to emotionally eat.

Some Common Feelings
Traumatized Children Experience

Guilt: Feeling responsible for something bad that happened to them or to someone else and believing it was their fault.

Shame and worthlessness: Feeling "not good enough," "bad," and like "damaged goods." Many people confuse guilt and shame. Think of it this way: Guilt is believing you did something "wrong" or "bad," while shame is believing *you* are "wrong" or "bad." Guilt judges an *action* (or inaction); shame judges *yourself*.

Loneliness: Stems from deep emotional isolation. This isn't necessarily about the child not having people in their life. It's about being unable to share their true emotions and experiences with these people.

Anger and rage: Think of anger and rage on a continuum. The child may express anger by talking or yelling and remain *somewhat* in control of their behavior. Rage, however, is harder to contain and can result in more aggressive behaviors. Both are responses to feeling helpless and powerless.

Helplessness: When children experience no control over inescapable trauma and learn that their actions are of no consequence, they may develop a state of "learned helplessness." In adulthood, this can result in passivity and low motivation to change oneself or one's environment.

Hopelessness: Often connected with helplessness, hopelessness arises from the realization that one cannot change a stressful or unsafe situation. The child emotionally collapses.

Sadness: May be chronic but with moments of happiness. With some traumatized children, you can see the sadness on their face. With others, it's hidden behind a plastic smile.

Fear: Knowing that something bad is happening or will inevitably happen, perhaps daily. Chronic fear may manifest as anxiety in the child's dysregulated body. Sometimes well-meaning professionals who lack trauma-informed skills may diagnose these symptoms as ADHD when they're actually signs of C-PTSD.

How are you doing? There's a lot of pain in this list, and it may be hard to read. Perhaps memories of yourself as a child or teen were triggered. If you need to take a break, please do so. Perhaps you can move your body—do some stretches, take a walk, use progressive muscle relaxation—or wrap yourself in your sacred shawl. Do whatever will be helpful to comfort and ground yourself. Come back when you're ready.

The Role of Adult Support

Children cannot process trauma-based feelings on their own. They need trusted adults to guide them. With family or professional help, they're then able to move through their feelings more easily. (No matter our age, we all benefit from having compassionate people in our life to process our feelings.) When children feel sad, angry, or scared and experience support, they learn that their feelings matter, hard feelings are okay, and they can move through them. For example:

- When a caring adult comforts a sad child, the child learns it's okay to feel sad and that sadness won't hurt them.

- When a supportive adult validates and helps the child verbalize anger, the child learns it's okay to feel angry and express it safely.

- When a loving adult reassures a scared child, the child learns how to move from fear to safety.

Many traumatized children, however, do not have the support they need to navigate their feelings. I imagine this was your experience too. When you were a child, the painful feelings listed above most likely could not be processed for these reasons:

- The adults in your life had good intentions but didn't know how to help you or believed you were okay because on the surface you appeared to function well.

- The trauma you experienced was hidden (as with sexual abuse), the adults in your life considered it non-problematic (as with denial around alcoholism), or they believed you "deserved" it (as with physical or emotional abuse).

Unprocessed feelings also weaken the child's intuition. Children learn they cannot trust their perception when they hear things like:

- "Don't be mad (or sad); it's better this way," when their parents divorce.

- "There's nothing wrong with your mother," when they see Mom acting strange from drinking too much wine.

- "Don't make up stories. Uncle Joey was just tickling you," when they try to disclose sexual abuse.

Or, they hear nothing at all.

It's hard to listen to your inner voice today when that voice wasn't heard in childhood. If this was your experience, I am so sorry that no one listened to your heart, and you felt such pain all by yourself. If you'd like, give yourself a warm hug with your sacred shawl and know that your Wise Self is with you always.

Let's now look more deeply at what happens to trauma-based feelings when they're unable to be processed in childhood.

It has been said that time heals all wounds, but that's not necessarily true. The abuse and trauma you experienced may have happened decades ago, but the passage of time doesn't matter because *feelings are timeless.* When feelings are not acknowledged, processed, and released, they remain frozen inside the mind and body. Your inner child doesn't know the difference between today and twenty or forty years ago. These painful feelings rule your life—and keep you turning to food—until you're able to acknowledge, feel, and heal them.

This is why, for many traumatized people, their reactions are out of proportion to the situation. For example, are you quick to anger at the slightest offense? Do you easily feel ashamed? Does rejection cripple you?

When you're feeling intense emotion, reflect on the possibility that what you're experiencing is a *memory* of what you felt a long time ago. We all hold visual memories. These are like photos you "see" in your mind. But feelings and emotions are memories too. You can't "see" them; you *feel* them in your body. And sometimes you feel them suddenly and intensely.

For example, Carol (from chapter 1) felt gripped with shame when she believed she made a mistake, said the "wrong thing" to coworkers, and especially, when she would emotionally eat. The shame she felt was real, but these present-day experiences triggered emotional memories from childhood. When painful feelings from the past reside within, you don't experience emotional stress in present time only. Your inner child and body are feeling both today's pain *and* the accumulation of unresolved pain. That's why your reaction may be out of proportion.

Healing and releasing trauma-based feelings allow your true self to emerge. That's the part of you that feels confident, self-trusting, and safe. (Yes. You *can* live your life this way.) It's okay that you've been using food for comfort when overwhelmed. That's not a sin. You've been doing the best you can. And I want you to know that underneath all that pain and sorrow is a core so strong, so loving, and so peaceful *that it can handle anything.*

This is your true self. She's still there, just waiting for you to find her.

How do you find her? By welcoming and feeling your feelings. *All of them.* The soft, gentle ones and the hard, overwhelming ones. Now I'll show you how.

Process Your Feelings Mindfully

This four-step process helps you mindfully meet your feelings, feel them, and integrate them into your mind, body, and spirit. The steps are:

1. Notice the feeling.

2. Name the feeling.

3. Accept the feeling.

4. Love the feeling.

We'll now address each step.

1. Notice the Feeling

This first step is developing awareness of what you're feeling in any moment. Perhaps you've used food to push away hard feelings and sensations for so long that you're not even sure what you feel or you experience intense trauma-based emotion that cripples you. Other times, whether you know what you feel or not, your feelings aren't getting in the way of daily life. Either way, you can learn the language of feelings by making a conscious choice to be mindful of how you feel throughout the day.

Let's start with this mini step: Several times a day, including right now, pause and ask yourself, "What am I feeling? What emotions am I experiencing?" Tune in to your body. What sensations do you notice, and where are they located? It's okay if you're not sure. Simply asking is the key to developing awareness.

Right before and after eating are important times to tune in to your body and ask yourself how you're feeling. This helps you develop awareness of how emotions and feelings relate to your food choices, portions, and emotional eating. You may want to write about this in your journal to notice connections between your feelings and eating.

2. Name the Feeling

When you're gripped with emotion and turn to food, you're unintentionally acting out your feelings. Acting-out children are taught to "use your words" instead of communicating through their behavior. Whether you're a child or an adult, this is effective because simply naming a feeling and saying it to yourself—I feel sad, I feel angry—activates the thinking part of your brain and helps you regain equilibrium. Imagine an attentive mother saying to her unhappy child, *"You look sad, honey."* The child feels safe knowing that someone sees them and understands. You can do the same for yourself—and your inner child.

Some feelings may be easier to identify than others. For example, you may know when you feel angry or worried. But it may be harder to identify when you feel sad or lonesome. That's because when feelings are unprocessed, it's hard to experience their variations along a broader spectrum.

Think of the color wheel. There are the primary colors of blue, red, and yellow. But the world is so much richer when you see the full range of color in the spectrum, right?

It's the same with your feelings. Your life is richer when you experience a range of feelings instead of being stuck in one or two default states. The more feelings you learn to experience, the more self-aware you become. You're then more in charge of your emotional life and, subsequently, more self-trusting.

Feelings can be identified within four primary categories with a spectrum of various shades. Review the following list when you're unsure about what you feel. It helps you identify and expand your palette of feelings. (You can download a copy of this list at http://www.newharbinger.com /51178.)

Sad   Lonely, disappointed, blue, unhappy, bored, dejected, guilty, ashamed, hurt, isolated, miserable, depressed, heartbroken, gloomy, despairing, grief, lonesome, hopeless, helpless, rejected, distressed, abandoned, alone, powerless, empty

Mad   Angry, frustrated, bitter, upset, annoyed, resentful, irritated, exasperated, loathing, disgusted, hostile, hateful, aggravated, defensive, enraged, livid, infuriated, irate, outraged, antagonistic, mean, indignation, furious, uncompromising, fuming

Glad   Happy, thankful, elated, delighted, cheerful, loving, hopeful, relief, appreciative, satisfied, excited, peaceful, enthusiastic, proud, pleased, caring, grateful, carefree, joyful, confident, secure, nurturing, content, blissful, ecstatic

Scared Anxious, nervous, panicky, afraid, worried, frightened, terrified, fearful, apprehensive, uneasy, concerned, insecure, vulnerable, weak, unsettled, tense, confused, upset, shocked, overwhelmed, suspicious, pressured, unsure, trapped, cautious

3. Accept the Feeling

Once you notice what you're feeling and can name it, it's time to *accept it.* You do this by saying the feeling out loud and telling yourself, "It's okay." Speak to yourself gently so your tone of voice offers nurturing comfort. For example:

"I feel lonely...and it's okay."

"I feel worried...and it's okay."

"I feel angry...and it's okay."

If you haven't been able to name what you're feeling, say to yourself: *"I don't know what I'm feeling...and it's okay."*

One feeling that is particularly hard to accept is shame. Humans naturally experience a healthy degree of shame (and guilt) to keep us from behaving badly toward others. But deep shame often is rooted in early trauma where the child internalized negative and false messages about their worth. This level of shame is emotionally debilitating. When triggered, accept the feeling in this way:

"I feel shame...and it's okay. It's just an old feeling I carry inside and is not the truth about who I am."

Saying "it's okay" doesn't mean it's not hard to feel a painful feeling. It means you accept that you are human, all your feelings have a reason for being there, and you can learn from them. So often we're given suggestions of what to "do" with our feelings. While that's important—I offer suggestions below—it's also important *to give ourselves reassurance and permission to feel.*

Your feelings cannot hurt you. It's what you *do* with them that either helps or hurts you, stifles self-growth, or harms others. So sometimes the best thing to do, at least at first is…nothing. Naming what you feel and learning to comfort yourself *with your own reassurance* empowers you. Do the best you can to allow your feelings to wash through your body, imagining them as waves of energy moving through and out of you.

Next, you'll take action.

4. Love It

How do you love hard feelings? The same way you'd love a crying baby or frustrated child. With tenderness, support, and reassurance. You never get to heal old wounds or experience the fullness of life if you mute your feelings with food. In the same way a distraught child needs comfort, your feelings need that tender approach too.

Below are strategies to soothe, release, and love your feelings in a safe way. (You can download a copy of the strategies at http://www.newharbinger.com/51178.) Each feeling category needs a different approach (although some overlap) because of how it's experienced in your body. Use this guide to discover what works best when you're feeling stressed and overwhelmed and, especially, when triggered to emotionally eat.

WHEN YOU FEEL SAD...COMFORT YOURSELF

Write your feelings in a journal. Call a friend. Have a good cry. Drink a cup of herbal tea. Read a book of inspirational quotes. Pray. Take a bath or shower. Wrap yourself in your sacred shawl. Add love to your sacred vessel. Take a nap. Work on a craft project. Listen to soothing music. Watch a sad movie to help release your feelings. Donate money to a favorite charity because giving to others uplifts our spirit. Affirm and reassure yourself: *"I feel sad and it's okay."*

WHEN YOU FEEL MAD...CALM YOURSELF

Breathe diaphragmatically to the count of ten and repeat until you feel calmer. Move your body to release tension, such as taking a brisk walk, vacuuming, or stretching. Listen to the "Peaceful Place" recording. Knit or crochet, which calms the mind and body. Find a detail-oriented activity to focus your mind, such as a word game, jigsaw puzzle, or coloring book. Write about the situation. Talk with a friend to gain perspective. Affirm and reassure yourself: *"I feel mad and it's okay."*

WHEN YOU FEEL GLAD...CELEBRATE YOURSELF

Write a letter of gratitude to your Wise Self. Call a friend to share your happiness. Buy yourself flowers. Buy flowers for a friend and spread the joy. Add love to your sacred vessel. Plan a solo or friend date to visit a museum or see a movie. Sit quietly by yourself in nature to relish this glorious state. Enjoy a hobby or craft that you don't take time to do. Affirm and appreciate: *"I feel glad and am grateful."*

WHEN YOU FEEL SCARED...GROUND YOURSELF

Unless your situation requires immediate attention, affirm and repeat, *"I am able to ground myself."* Breathe diaphragmatically to the count of ten and repeat until you feel calmer. Sit with both feet firmly on the floor with your back straight, breathing steadily until you feel centered. Look around and name ten things that you see. Do something physical to release tension from your body: Walk, vacuum, wash floors. Clear clutter from a drawer because organizing your outer world helps organize your inner world. Talk with a friend to put things in perspective. *Affirm and reassure yourself:* "I feel scared and it's okay."

Now that you've learned strategies to use with different categories of feelings, here's the fun part.

Create Your Self-Care Basket

Find a pretty basket or box. Then, drawing from the suggestions above and below, or from what has helped in the past, write a list of objects and activities that help you create a soothing experience, healthy distraction, or relaxing environment. Think of these as your happiness triggers.

Here are ten suggestions of items to put in your self-care basket:

- aromatherapy candle

- herbal teas

- knitting, crafts, or art materials

- journal and pen

- playlist of your favorite music

- coloring book and pencils

- word-puzzle book

- book of daily inspiration or prayers

- anti-stress squeeze ball

- list of people to call for support

Gather the items and put them in your basket. You've now created a go-to resource for self-soothing and comfort. Overwhelm clouds the mind. Your self-care basket offers support without having to think about what can help.

Instead of turning to food, turn to your basket.

When experiencing a hard feeling, choose an item. Knowing you have a collection of resources helps reassure you and your inner child that self-soothing—without turning to food—is possible.

While your self-care basket will help in times of stress, I'd like you to use it *all the time* so happiness triggers become a normal part of your daily life. Give yourself "me-time" today or this week to create your self-care basket because *you and your feelings are worth it.*

The Power of Pausing

Now that you've learned the four steps to mindfully process your feelings, I'm going to teach you a neuroscience rule that can be a game changer to help you take charge of particularly overwhelming emotions. It's called the Ninety-Second Rule, and I learned about it from Jill Bolte Taylor (2006, 146), PhD, in her book *My Stroke of Insight: A Brain Scientist's Personal Journey*: "Although there are certain limbic system (emotional) programs that can be triggered automatically, it takes less than ninety seconds for one of these programs to be triggered, surge through our body, and then be completely flushed out of our bloodstream."

This means that once you feel triggered with overwhelming emotion, *it takes just ninety seconds for the stress you feel to leave your body.* After that, you're in charge. You either keep the stress response active with fear-based thoughts or can mindfully allow your body to calm down.

This is powerful information. In earlier chapters, you learned about the body's stress response. What's liberating about the Ninety-Second Rule is that it gives you confidence to pause when triggered because you know your body's stress response will eventually wash out of your system. When you keep thinking stressful thoughts, you're unintentionally restimulating the emotional circuitry that keeps the stress response activated.

For example, if you're triggered after an argument with your mother and keep ruminating over angry thoughts, your body stays dysregulated. You're then susceptible to using food to ground yourself. But when you're able to *pause and bring your mind to neutral* for ninety seconds, your body has a chance to settle down. Now, I'm not saying this is easy to do. I sometimes find it impossible to quiet my own monkey-mind. But the good news is we now know that when we quiet that chatter, our bodies have a chance to recover. This helps you respond mindfully, rather than impulsively, to hard feelings.

Here's what I want you to do: When you feel triggered with overwhelming emotion and it's too hard to follow step 1 above and simply notice, say to yourself, "ninety seconds." Then, breathe diaphragmatically for a couple of minutes to allow the emotion to move through and out of your body. Adding structure helps focus your mind to get to that neutral place. For example, while breathing:

- Count each exhale.

- With eyes open or closed, focus on your right big toe. You can focus on anything really, but your big toe is always with you and most likely a neutral part of your body.

- Focus your mind on something loved or beautiful. For example, your child's face, relaxing at the beach, or your favorite flower.

Once your body settles, you're in a better position to deal with the situation and the feelings triggered.

Sometimes the Ninety-Second Rule will help; other times it may seem impossible to stop your thoughts from hijacking your mind. That's okay. Think progress, not perfection.

A Bridge to Healing

As you learned, unprocessed feelings are timeless. The pain cuts deep and can be overwhelming. One way to heal unprocessed childhood pain at its deep level is to link today's pain with its original source.

Early in my career, I learned a hypnosis technique called the "affect bridge," which was developed by psychologist John G. Watkins (1971) in the early 1970s. I've adapted this strategy in my work with clients and call it the "feeling bridge." I use the feeling bridge to explore the connection between emotional reactions today and their roots in the past.

For example, do you feel shame after making a simple mistake, like Carol does? Do you react with anger at the slightest inconvenience? When friends don't return a call, does it trigger abandonment?

Your reaction isn't only about a present time event but is the aftershock from an earlier earthquake. Once you heal from the earthquake, you either don't get the aftershocks or, if you do, they're mild.

The feeling bridge is a writing and visualization exercise to explore the root cause of why you're hypersensitive in certain situations. This isn't a coping strategy. It's a process to help heal your inner child. You can use the feeling bridge shortly after a strong emotion hits or after some time has passed. But when you do this the first few times, practice with an emotional reaction that no longer feels raw. After you're comfortable using the feeling bridge, you'll know the best time to safely practice.

The Feeling Bridge

You may want to wear your sacred shawl when you practice the feeling bridge exercise. That way, you can feel secure in the arms of your Wise Self as you explore your inner child's feelings. Have your journal handy and settle yourself in a quiet, comfortable place where you won't be disturbed for about one hour.

After you've regrouped from having experienced strong emotion, journal on the following questions.

- What was I feeling, and what triggered it?

- How familiar is this feeling?

- When have I felt this way before?

After journaling on the above questions, ask yourself: "What is my first memory of feeling this way?"

Then, close your eyes and focus on the feeling to a tolerable degree. As if you're traveling back in time along a bridge of this feeling, gently allow images to enter your mind of the earliest times in your life when you felt this way. Trust that you're ready to see whatever images emerge. If you see several, allow your mind to settle on one. Stay there a moment. Breathe. Then open your eyes and journal about what you remembered.

Most intense, recurring emotions stem from childhood or adolescence. But if the image that entered your mind was from a previous experience in your adult life, journal on that. Most likely, repeated practice of using the feeling bridge will bring you back to an earlier time (unless the core trauma you experienced was from adulthood). If no images entered your mind, that's okay. Perhaps you're not yet ready to explore this and can practice later.

Now, close your eyes again and call up the image of you as that child or adolescent and imagine the adult you and your child (or teen) together in a cozy space. Visualize yourself telling her that you're sorry she went through such pain and that you're going to take care of her. If you feel comfortable, imagine giving her a hug. Stay with the image as long as you like. Then, open your eyes and notice what it was like to give comfort and support to your child within.

Journal on this experience.

The feeling bridge exercise helps you connect with the true source of your pain to give your inner child the comfort she didn't receive long ago.

Carol practiced the feeling bridge to explore the root cause of why she easily felt shame. Her mind settled on a memory of her mother criticizing her body in front of classmates. Carol recalled how humiliated she felt. Through imagery, she connected with her inner twelve-year-old and offered her love and reassurance. Carol also hugged herself with her sacred shawl and added love to her sacred vessel when shame-filled beliefs entered her mind. These practices helped Carol soothe the root cause of shame.

While still triggered at times, she was better able to "be with" feelings of shame instead of numbing them with food.

Putting It All Together

We've covered a lot in this chapter, and some sections may have triggered difficult memories—for you *and* your inner child. It's not easy to revisit painful childhood feelings, so be gentle and nurturing with yourself.

Learning to notice, name, accept, and treat your feelings lovingly will transform your life. You've probably spent years pushing away hard feelings with food, so it will take time to unlearn that and embrace a new path. By following the four steps, creating your self-care basket, using the Ninety-Second Rule, and traveling the feeling bridge, over time you'll begin to process and relate to your feelings in a nurturing way. As that happens, your impulse to use food to cope will lessen. And even if the urge doesn't subside completely, that's okay. You're developing self-awareness, self-trust, and self-compassion—and reconnecting with your true self. That's what it means to heal, and ultimately, what matters most.

Now that you've learned how to nurture a peaceful relationship with your feelings, in the next chapter you'll learn how to make peace with food.

CHAPTER 7

Take Your Power Back from Trigger Foods

Emotional eating and dieting often are closely connected behaviors. I wonder if this is your experience too. Maybe you've ridden the yo-yo-diet roller coaster with its restrictive rules and rigid approach to food. Diet culture can wreak havoc on your relationship with foods, your body, and mostly, your relationship with yourself. When you're told by supposed authorities what, when, and how much you "can" and "cannot" eat, you lose touch with your innate sense of what's best for you and your body. Learning about sound nutrition and the effects of certain foods on your particular health needs is important. But otherwise, trust that only you and your body know what foods and in what proportions are best for your optimal well-being.

Years of dieting, especially if you were put on diets when you were a child, can distort and undermine your relationship with food. Food becomes tension-filled when some are deemed off-limits or "bad." It's easy to then judge yourself as "bad" for eating them and "good" when you don't. When you've experienced childhood trauma and hold within feelings of worthlessness, you may be especially triggered to feel "bad" for eating a certain food. Diet culture promotes this attitude, so even people who did not experience early trauma may judge their self-worth by their food choices. But when childhood trauma is not yet healed and you're already filled with underlying guilt and shame, you're even more susceptible to getting caught in the clutches of diet culture's judgments. Remember what you learned in chapter 6 about feelings being timeless? The guilt and shame you feel for eating what you judge as a "bad" food can trigger underlying guilt and shame that are already inside of you. It's then not only about the food. It's about your deeper sense of worth. Do you really want to give *any* food that kind of power over you?

Food is neutral. It's the meaning we give it that matters. While neutral, it's also true that different foods offer our bodies varied nutritional support. We know that fresh whole foods are more healthful than ultra-processed foods. I'm not a dietitian or in the food industry business, so it's beyond the scope of my expertise to address nutrition or the production and marketing of food. I will assume that if you're reading this book, you've probably dieted, are aware of healthy nutrition, and know at least some (good and questionable) practices of our food industry.

And no matter what some diet says, I hope you know that it's okay to eat cookies. Including packaged ones. When you believe you "cannot" eat a food that you enjoy, that food paradoxically may become even more appealing to you. There's a popular saying (often attributed to psychiatrist Carl Jung) that suggests, "What you resist not only persists, but will grow in size." (You're probably familiar with the simplified version, "What you resist, persists.") That's what happens when you believe you "cannot" eat a food that you enjoy and want to eat. Restrictive diets encourage you to "resist" that food, which then can create obsessive thoughts about that food, which "persist." These obsessive thoughts then can lead to eating that food, often in large proportions, as a reaction against the restriction. Trauma survivors who experienced emotional or physical deprivation may feel the effects of restriction especially acutely due to the unprocessed pain carried within.

Giving yourself permission to eat what you want and "legalizing" food is a concept popularized in the 1980s by Susie Orbach (1982), author of *Fat Is a Feminist Issue II: A Program to Conquer Compulsive Eating;*

psychotherapist Jane Hirschmann and psychoanalyst Carol Munter (1988) in their book *Overcoming Overeating: How to Break the Diet/Binge Cycle and Live a Healthier, More Satisfying Life;* and Geneen Roth (1984), author of *Breaking Free from Emotional Eating.* These authors encouraged readers to purchase all the foods they wanted to eat that they previously forbade themselves from eating. This wasn't a one-time shopping experience but the beginning step toward a balanced relationship with food. Making peace with food by "legalizing" it also is endorsed by registered dietitians Evelyn Tribole and Elyse Resch (2020) in their bestselling book, *Intuitive Eating: A Revolutionary Anti-Diet Approach.* Their approach also is a freedom-filled contrast to the rigid constraints of diet culture.

Legalizing all foods helps you create an empowered mindset. Once you say no to diet culture with its "should not's" and "cant's," you're free to *intuitively learn* what you and your body desire. Following a rigid diet plan disconnects you from your body's needs, while legalizing food puts you in charge of your choices. Instead of relying on a diet to tell you what, how much, and when to eat, you rely on *yourself* in partnership with your body.

Allowing yourself to eat foods you truly want while honoring your body's hunger-fullness needs, validates your self-worth. No one but *you* know what foods you desire. When you restrict your choices due to diet culture, you're dishonoring yourself. Our food choices and body's needs are intensely personal. Abandoning that choice undermines your self-worth. But as you learn to eat freely, you gain self-agency. As a victim of childhood trauma, you most likely had little control over your early life. But you're no longer a child, and making food choices that align with your desires is an act of autonomy and self-respect. If you want a cheeseburger, eat one. If you want a salad, eat one. This doesn't mean you disregard your health needs. If you have medical issues requiring dietary vigilance, of course that's important to follow. As you honor what you and your body need and heed your hunger-fullness levels, you're supporting your body to reach its optimal level of wellness.

Gaining self-agency—especially around the food you give your body—is another aspect of healing. Legalizing food, respecting your body's needs, and making free choices about what you eat are important steps not only toward making peace with food but also toward *making peace with yourself.* You're in charge of your life. No one else. And certainly not some rigid diet plan.

All the clients I have seen over the years for emotional eating were also traumatized as children or adolescents. Perhaps this is due to my having an expertise in childhood trauma, so many clients come to me for that reason. Or perhaps it's due to screening for childhood trauma when I begin meeting with a client and we discover issues the client may not have interpreted as affecting their life and relationship with food. Whatever the reason, I have not worked with anyone for whom emotional eating stemmed from the effects of diet culture only. While not everyone affected by diet culture experienced childhood trauma, having a trauma history exacerbates the damaging effects of diet culture and needs to be acknowledged and addressed for sustained change to happen.

When I started working with traumatized clients who had spent years dieting, I too, endorsed legalizing all foods. It's a powerful mind-shift for people who normally restrict what they eat. However, I found that while this approach helped many people, it didn't help everyone. Sharon helped me realize that there simply isn't a one-size-fits-all approach to food (or most things).

A thirty-nine-year-old nurse, Sharon began therapy shortly after her mother died of alcoholism. Overcome with grief, Sharon was surprised at how her mother's death affected her. Three years earlier, she had ended contact because she no longer would tolerate her mother's abusive behavior.

Sharon's history revealed a childhood of emotional and physical abuse, alcoholism, and domestic violence. Both of her parents drank excessively. She described her father as a depressed man who "drowned his sorrow in vodka" and her mother as a mean-spirited woman who physically abused her and her father. "It was a toxic home environment," she said, "and I did what I could do to protect my younger siblings."

When I asked what helped her cope, Sharon said she found comfort in food. "After my parents' hideous fights, my father would pass out in his chair, and my mother would get lost in television and a bottle of wine. I'd put my brother and sister to sleep and then sit in my room watching TV and eating chips and candy until I stopped feeling anything. I think food numbed me out."

"My mother was beautiful," Sharon said. "I never could measure up. She put me on my first diet when I was eight. She didn't treat my brother and sister this way, but she was obsessed with how I looked. I remember how ashamed I felt when she would give my siblings dessert but say I couldn't have any.

"I rebelled against dieting—and my mother—by stealing money from her purse to buy snacks from the store. Then, in my mid-teens I got obsessed with my weight and dieting. That's when I stopped using food so much and began drinking."

Leaving home for college was a lifesaver for Sharon. After a binge-drinking episode that resulted in a fall down her dorm staircase, her resident advisor encouraged her to see a school counselor. Therapy helped Sharon stop drinking, and she started attending Alcoholics Anonymous meetings. She said that once she quit drinking, she began emotionally eating again. Therapy had helped with Sharon's alcohol addiction—and this was a huge accomplishment—but it did not address early trauma. While she eliminated alcohol from her life, she could not eliminate the deeper pain. Food replaced wine as her main way to cope.

The grief Sharon felt about her mother's death, which prompted her to start therapy again, triggered pain from childhood trauma and intensified emotional eating. Even though she broke off contact, she secretly wished her mother would change. "I was always hoping for that one phone call from her saying, 'I'm sorry I hurt you.' Of course, that call never came. And then the call came that she died."

A self-aware woman, Sharon was motivated to create positive change in her life. Our work together helped her grieve the loving mother she never had. Psychotherapy needs to be paced, so when Sharon was ready, we then addressed emotional eating and her relationship with food and her body. Knowing my approach did not endorse diets, Sharon was open to creating a more balanced relationship with food and getting off the yo-yo-diet roller coaster. She had had enough.

Sharon's history of childhood and adult dieting skewed her relationship with food. She was stuck in seeing herself as "bad" if she ate sweets or pasta and "good" if she ate vegetables. Much of our work addressed separating her self-worth from what she ate and healing the shame and self-loathing she carried from childhood. She was open to legalizing all foods and allowed herself to eat what she wanted to eat.

An area of continued struggle, however, was with certain foods, specifically chips and candy bars, which Sharon would compulsively eat once she started. These foods offered comfort when she was growing up, and she wanted to enjoy them. But no matter how much Sharon tried to eat these mindfully, she couldn't stop overeating them in ways that felt physically uncomfortable. She hadn't yet learned how to comfort herself without using food, and legalizing chips and candy bars didn't stop her from using them to cope when she was upset. In one of our sessions, she said that she didn't think she could keep buying these foods. When I suggested that she again use mindful-eating skills, she said, "Diane—I love working with you, but I don't think you get it. In the same way I couldn't mindfully sip wine without overdoing it, I cannot mindfully eat candy bars and chips without overdoing it. For me, it's the same thing."

Sharon was right. She called me out on my one-size-fits-all approach based on what I had read but without enough years of experience to be nuanced with it. She didn't think she would feel deprived if she stopped buying chips and candy—even though a part of her wanted to eat them—and decided it was best to no longer keep them at home. "On the contrary," she said. "I'm not depriving myself. I think I'm taking care of myself."

For Sharon, candy bars and chips were trigger foods. "Trigger foods" is a term used to describe foods that you can't easily stop eating once you start. Common trigger foods include foods high in salt, fats, refined carbs, or sugar, such as potato chips, ice cream, pasta, bread, and cookies. I want to emphasize that *food is neutral*, and there is nothing wrong or bad about eating these foods. (I'm Italian and was raised on pasta!) It's about how *you* respond to these and other foods.

For some people, even those who don't eat for emotional reasons, a trigger food itself induces a craving to eat it. For example, you see the bag of chips and dig in, and it has nothing to do with how you feel or whether you're hungry. For other people, eating a trigger food is their way to cope when they feel emotionally triggered. Even though Sharon ultimately chose to stop bringing candy bars and chips home, she would eat them occasionally at a restaurant or party. When she was feeling overwhelmed and nothing else worked to help her feel better, she would drive to the store and buy them. The breakthrough for Sharon was that she learned how to be kind to herself and stopped beating herself up when she did this. Even though emotional overwhelm sometimes triggered her to eat candy bars and chips, she still preferred to keep them out of her home. She said, "Even though I sometimes feel compelled to buy them, out of sight is best for me. Otherwise, I'd devour them, and I don't want to do that." For Sharon, emotionally eating chips and candy bars didn't stop when she "legalized" them. That's because she believed it was another form of addiction, much like drinking alcohol had been.

There is debate about what constitutes a true addiction. I'm not a researcher and will not dive into those waters. As a clinical psychotherapist, however, I know that certain substances (food, alcohol, other drugs) and behaviors (shopping, gambling, sex) can hold emotional power over people and serve as tools for self-medicating because, in part, they activate the reward centers in our brain. For example, even the anticipation of eating a trigger food (or buying a new pair of shoes) can produce a calming effect that offers a bit of relief in the space between feeling overwhelmed and being able to access and eat that food (or buy those heels). Is this a true addiction? I don't know, but for the purposes of helping my clients, it doesn't matter how I label it. Helping them learn to calm their nervous system and attend to their feelings in self-loving ways, as you've been learning, is key—no matter what term I use to describe their relationship with certain foods.

JOURNAL PROMPTS

Reflect on the following questions and journal on what comes up for you.

- Are there foods you enjoy that fit the description of trigger foods? If so, write them down.

- Do you eat these foods when you feel emotionally overwhelmed? When you're feeling content and see these foods, are they hard to resist?

- Thinking of each food, what happens once you start eating it? How can you tell when your body has had enough of that food? Can you stop eating once you reach a level of physical satisfaction? Or is it hard to stop?

- If it's hard to stop, journal on why you feel compelled to keep eating. Is it the taste of the food? Is it the way the food calms your emotions? Are you unsure?

- If you've tried to mindfully eat these foods, what happened?

- Do you buy and keep these foods at home? Or, like Sharon, do you prefer to not buy them? Either way, how does your choice help you?

My work with Sharon helped me realize that encouraging my clients to legalize all food without appropriate boundaries specific to their needs was not necessarily helpful. My job was to offer flexibility so they could discover what worked best for them and their body. You can discover what works best for you too.

Let's start by reframing your relationship with trigger foods. Think about it. There are reasons why people restrict their food choices that have nothing to do with diet culture, and saying no to those foods doesn't necessarily induce the urge to eat them. For example, if you have celiac disease, it's critical to stay away from gluten. With certain diseases and sensitivities, there are limits to legalizing all food. Many people navigate this successfully, and sometimes unsuccessfully, but they don't feel "deprived." Knowing they "cannot" have certain foods—even foods they love—doesn't necessarily cause them to obsess about it. In contrast to the restrictions of diet culture, in these situations, choosing to avoid the food doesn't create a persistent desire for it. The difference is in your mindset and *believing you're making a conscious and free choice.*

What made the difference for Sharon was thinking about the word "deprived" differently. Our words are powerful. They create our beliefs, inform our actions, and have the power to activate or calm our nervous system. As a child on restrictive diets, and especially having to watch her siblings eat desserts she wasn't allowed to have, Sharon *did* feel deprived. This emotional abuse, coupled with the other trauma she experienced at home, exacerbated feelings of deprivation, shame, and worthlessness. As an adult, the restrictive diets Sharon followed reinforced her feelings of deprivation. While your early experience may have been different from Sharon's, perhaps you can relate to her challenges. (And, as always, if you're feeling triggered, remember to breathe diaphragmatically, take a break, and give yourself a hug with your sacred shawl.)

Legalizing food helped Sharon immensely. While she eventually chose to not bring certain foods home, this new approach to foods felt liberating and changed her thinking. For the first time in her life, she felt free to eat the way she wanted to eat. As Sharon began to think differently about food and the words "deprived," "can't," and "shouldn't," she felt more empowered, and paradoxically, she stopped bringing certain foods into her home. Her thinking changed in these two powerful ways:

She stopped associating the word "deprived" with food. (Sadly, this is not possible for people who experience food insecurity. If this is your reality, I am so sorry that you're struggling and hope you find resources in your community to help you.) When feelings of deprivation would get triggered for Sharon, either around food she chose not to eat or by life stress, she understood that this pain had nothing to do with food but was connected to the *emotional* deprivation she experienced as a child. She said, "Real deprivation is having no food to eat or water to drink. I won't let myself feel deprived just because I choose not to eat a candy bar." Recognizing the root cause of feeling deprived—and healing on that level—was key in helping Sharon heal her relationship with food.

The word "can't" regarding food took on a lighter meaning. She said, "I can't have candy bars or chips in the house, and that's not because some diet is telling me not to. It's because they're too tempting and once I start eating them, I can't seem to stop. I'm not denying myself. I'm *choosing* not to bring them home, and that's okay. It doesn't make me want them more. Even when I feel stressed and sometimes run out to buy them, I prefer to do that. Plus, I'm better able to ground myself so that doesn't happen so much anymore."

Your Choice

How you relate to trigger foods helps you create peace or keeps you in constant struggle. Take time to decide how you want to approach them. I offer you two choices to consider. One choice is to not bring trigger foods home and possibly to avoid eating them altogether. The other choice is to buy them to have available at home.

What's most important is that you make a *conscious choice* rooted in what you believe is *best for you and your body* and unrelated to diet culture or what works for someone else.

Choosing to Avoid Trigger Foods

Some people avoid trigger foods completely. For others, there's flexibility. For example, you may choose not to bring certain foods home but decide to eat them at a party or restaurant. If you choose this approach, reflect on these questions:

- Will feelings of deprivation be triggered if you don't eat these foods? If so, how confident do you feel in your ability to soothe and comfort yourself with these feelings?

- If feelings of deprivation get triggered, will that cause you to eat the food in a way that feels uncomfortable for your body? If so, how confident do you feel in your ability to not judge yourself or feel guilty?

- How will you handle it if family members bring these foods home?

- How do you believe keeping trigger foods out of your home will be helpful to you?

There is great freedom in taking a stand against something that you believe causes you harm or confusion. Those who make this choice successfully keep an empowered mindset. Instead of thinking they "cannot" eat these foods, they "choose" not to eat them. Instead of believing they're "denying" themselves, they believe they're taking good care of themselves.

Choosing to Allow Trigger Foods

Some people choose to buy and eat all foods they enjoy eating. This helps them break free from a self-depriving notion that they "should not" or "cannot" eat certain foods. As you learned, when you "legalize" all foods and remove restrictions, you liberate yourself from the tension surrounding these foods and from the rigid constraints of diet culture. If you choose this approach, reflect on these questions:

- Will you be able to mindfully satisfy a desire or craving with a reasonable portion? If so, what helps you feel confident about this?

- Will you be triggered to emotionally eat these foods when stressed? If so, how confident do you feel in your ability to not judge yourself?

- How do you believe keeping these foods available at home will be helpful to you?

It's sometimes easier to set boundaries on our behavior when we feel we have choice. If you allow yourself to eat these foods, you may experience a freedom that, paradoxically, minimizes your desire.

Journal on the reflection questions above to decide how you want to relate to trigger foods and what option will work best for you. You may also want to connect with and ask your Wise Self for guidance. I've included a question in the "Meet Your Wise Self" audio to help you feel at peace with food (available at http://www.newharbinger.com/51178).

A Word About Mindful Eating

Simply put, mindful eating is the ability to focus on the food you're eating without clouding your mind with external distractions or ruminative thoughts. You're aware of your emotional state before, during, and after eating. You feel attuned to your body's signs of hunger, fullness, and satisfaction before, during, and after eating. You're not rushing but eating slowly enough to savor and enjoy your food. There are many great books on mindful eating, and I've listed some of my favorites in the "Resources" section.

Now, I agree with almost everything about mindful eating, but I do believe this: it's okay to eat a meal while watching television.

For some people, especially trauma survivors who live alone, having a television on in the background is a form of human contact. Obviously, it's not the same as being with someone. But if you struggle with loneliness, you may feel a little less lonely hearing people talk and seeing them interact. And as Carol said in chapter 1, *"When it gets quiet on the outside, it gets real noisy on the inside."* It's then easy to shift to emotional eating when a quiet home triggers inner turmoil. Watching a favorite show or movie is also a way to destress. If watching television offers you support while eating a meal, it's okay. I think you can eat and watch TV at the same time *if* you do it mindfully and stay attuned to your body's hunger-fullness levels. In terms of distractions, it's similar to being at a restaurant with friends or at a dinner party. In those situations, there are lots of distractions too, yet people can still mindfully eat *and* talk and interact.

I do caution you against using social media while eating. Looking at YouTube, Instagram, or Facebook can lead you down the cyber rabbit hole. You're then interacting with the device versus passively watching a television show at a distance while mindfully enjoying dinner.

If you have children, I suggest you keep devices away from the table entirely. Mealtimes are important opportunities for bonding, and screens get in the way of that. If you live with a partner or roommate only and enjoy having dinner together while watching television (and not looking at another screen), that's fine and just do your best to eat slowly and mindfully.

Season Your Food with Love

As you create a peaceful relationship with food, here's a beautiful practice to help you along the way: add a pinch of love and gratitude.

You probably use salt and pepper shakers, right? A love-and-gratitude shaker is the same thing. But instead of enhancing the taste of your food, you're enhancing your relationship. Adding love and gratitude to any relationship makes that relationship stronger and more intimate. It's the same with food. Here's what you do:

- Buy or use a shaker you already own that you designate for this purpose. It could be a simple one made of glass or delicate porcelain, whatever resonates with you.

- Then, lovingly hold the shaker in your hands, close your eyes, and connect with your Wise Self.

- Say out loud or silently, "Dear Wise Self, please fill this shaker with infinite love and gratitude." Then, imagine a golden light pouring down from above filling your shaker with this beautiful energy.

- Stay quietly for a moment holding your shaker. Then, say, "Thank you," and open your eyes.

You don't need to repeat this because once you add love and gratitude to your shaker, it's filled forever.

With every meal or snack, use your shaker to add love and gratitude to your food before eating. If you traditionally say grace, using your shaker can add to that practice.

Be intentional. Pause, pick up your shaker, and imagine adding the energy of love and gratitude to your food while saying to yourself, "Love and gratitude." Thank the food for how it will give your body nutrients and the sensation of good taste. You may also want to offer thanks to the people who helped bring this food to you, for example, farm workers, truckers, retail employees. If you live with others and they want some of these sacred ingredients, pass the shaker around. If they don't, use it for yourself only. You also may wish to make two love-and-gratitude shakers. One to keep home and one to take with you when eating out.

Use your shaker *every time you eat*. This is important because your love-and-gratitude shaker isn't only for when you're eating peacefully. It's also to be used when you're feeling overwhelmed and triggered to emotionally eat. Sharon found that using her love-and-gratitude shaker often helped calm her. She said, "Taking a moment to pause and add love and gratitude to candy bars when I'm upset helps me be less judgmental of myself. It doesn't necessarily stop me from eating, but that's okay. It helps me slow down and be mindful of what I'm doing even when I'm overwhelmed and using food to cope."

How do you think a love-and-gratitude shaker will help you and your relationship with food, especially when you eat to soothe yourself? Perhaps you'd like to find a shaker this week and get started. A sprinkle of love and gratitude might add the comforting touch you need.

Putting It All Together

When you eat for emotional reasons, discussing your relationship with food can feel unsettling and confusing. Writing can create clarity, so take time to journal on what has come up for you while reading this chapter. Answer the prompts and reflect on what trigger foods mean to you, the kind of relationship you want to have, and what approach will best work for you, your body, and your unique needs.

As you heal from childhood trauma, develop new ways to soothe overwhelming feelings, and learn to think about trigger foods differently, your relationship with these foods will change. You may choose to no longer eat them, or you may still enjoy them, but you'll no longer feel tension around them. This journey takes time, so have patience. Eventually, your struggle with *all* food will lessen to the point that *you* feel in charge of your food choices instead of food taking charge of you.

And remember to season your food with love and gratitude, mindfully and always.

We'll now continue to the next chapter, where you'll learn about the true antidote to healing emotional eating—self-compassion.

CHAPTER 8

Transform Self-Punishment into Self-Compassion

How are you doing? We've addressed some hard issues thus far, and I imagine it's a lot to process. Pace yourself and take time to integrate it all. You've learned how to calm your nervous system; how to connect with your body; practices to acknowledge, release, *and love* your feelings and subconscious beliefs; and how to make peace with foods that hold power over you. These skills will not only help you heal emotional eating, but they'll also help you heal from childhood trauma too.

Now I'm going to share something about emotional eating that sounds counterintuitive but is important for you to understand: **Ending emotional eating isn't about *not* emotionally eating. It's about how you handle it when you do.**

I bet this sounds strange. You're reading this book because you want to *stop* emotional eating. But I ask you to put this goal aside because, for a while, you probably will emotionally eat.

And that's okay.

I'm not suggesting that you give yourself carte blanche permission to eat in a way that will hurt you or your body. I'm suggesting that you treat yourself with tenderness and compassion when you do.

Think of it this way: Even people who don't struggle with emotional eating sometimes overeat or eat when stressed. Most everyone does at times. They may feel uncomfortable afterward and wish they hadn't eaten so much, but they don't beat themselves up for it. They feel no guilt, shame, or remorse. So they can let it go.

And you can learn to let it go too.

For example, instead of scolding yourself for eating a whole pizza because you were upset with your partner, you accept you ate it and let it go. Instead of drowning yourself in guilt for eating a tub of ice cream because you felt lonely on Saturday night, you accept you slipped into a familiar habit and let it go. Instead of hating yourself for driving to the nearest drive-through for a burger and fries—after eating dinner—you accept you ate a second meal and let it go.

You may be thinking, *Diane, what are you talking about? Why should I accept a habit I want to stop?*

Let me explain. Remember what you learned in chapter 7 that "what you resist not only persists, but will grow in size"? When you expend energy fighting against something—and berating yourself for eating is fighting a habit you want to stop—you give emotional eating power over you. And beating yourself up also keeps you living in a painful past.

It's time to end the self-abuse.

It's hard—impossible, really—to overcome emotional eating by using harsh, self-critical words. Emotional eating gains momentum and "grows in size" each time you beat yourself up.

Heal it—and you—with kindness instead.

The Healing Power of Self-Compassion

Self-compassion is a powerful and proven practice to calm your nervous system, soothe your feelings, and rewire your brain to shift from disempowering, trauma-based beliefs to self-loving beliefs. As you learned in chapter 3, Dr. Kristin Neff (2011) is a pioneer in the field of self-compassion research and author of *Self-Compassion: The Proven Power of Being Kind to Yourself*. She notes how self-compassion and self-kindness are not "feel good" notions without substance. They are rooted in science and activate your body's mammalian care-giving system to release the hormone oxytocin. Oxytocin is considered the hormone of love and bonding, not only for others but also for ourselves. When you attack yourself with harsh, critical thoughts and words, your brain's amygdala and stress response are activated. As far as your brain is concerned, a threat from others or a threat from yourself is the same. Self-compassion practices help calm your amygdala and release oxytocin to help you feel soothed—even when you're the one attacking you.

You truly hold the power to heal yourself. The self-compassion practices in this chapter (and book) help you unlock that power.

The road to freedom from emotional eating is smoother when it's paved with self-love and kindness. This means that instead of criticizing yourself after you eat, you give yourself reassurance, tenderness, and compassion.

Developing Gentler Self-Talk

Quitting emotional eating cold turkey isn't realistic, but developing gentler, compassionate self-talk is. Read these words silently or out loud and let them sink into your body and soul: "When I emotionally eat, I will nourish myself with kind words and tenderness."

Now, close your eyes, breathe, and repeat the sentence while noticing the sensations in your body.

What did it feel like to say this? What sensations did you notice in your body? My clients often report a calming sensation when they say these self-compassionate words and feel more confident and hopeful. Others feel tension around these words because they don't believe them. If you experience tension, confusion, or other hard feelings, that's okay. Developing your self-compassion muscle takes practice. Trust that, over time, these words of kindness will become your new truth.

Saying "when I emotionally eat" doesn't mean you're reinforcing a habit you want to stop. It acknowledges where you are today while shining a light forward. And saying "I will nourish myself with kind words and tenderness" affirms you're becoming someone who treats themselves lovingly. Remember, even people who do not struggle with emotional eating sometimes eat when stressed. This affirmation reflects how they naturally let it go.

Meet Pain with Tenderness

In his bestselling book *The Power of Now: A Guide to Spiritual Enlightenment,* Eckhart Tolle (1999, 127) says, "Every addiction arises from an unconscious refusal to face and move through your own pain." In other words, addiction is a way to suppress emotional pain, whether you're addicted to food, alcohol, other drugs, sex, or shopping. Tolle also says that addictive behavior not only starts with pain, but it also ends with pain. For example, the pain that starts an emotional eating episode often ends with guilt and shame. It's a pain-propelled feedback loop of trauma-based beliefs and feelings. You may know it well.

As I mentioned earlier, there are mixed opinions about whether emotional eating is an addiction or compulsive behavior triggered by an emotional need. Semantics aside, you know when you feel overwhelming emotion and unsettling sensations in your body. You feel the urge to eat as a way to cope. You grab the nearest candy bar, box of cookies, or fast food to numb your pain—or plan a time to binge later.

Then, rather than accepting that you ate and dealing with what triggered you, you beat yourself up for eating. Fueled by harsh self-talk, the pain persists and "grows in size," and you feel worse.

What started in pain ends in pain.

The pain you feel for eating—guilt, self-loathing, shame—most likely is rooted in the trauma you experienced as a child. It also may be intertwined with years of restrictive dieting, especially if you were put on diets in childhood or adolescence. But I want you to understand that you're not experiencing these feelings just because you ate. *These feelings already are inside of you.* Emotional eating brings them to the surface. Let's review again why.

In chapter 6, you learned how feelings are timeless and that early trauma-based emotions remain inside your mind and body until they are processed and released. This makes it hard to stop emotionally eating because, once triggered, the pain you experienced ten, twenty, or forty, years ago becomes alive today. For example:

- Guilt about eating stimulates the deeper guilt that you—and your inner child—carry from believing what happened to you was your fault.

- Shame for eating heightens the deeper shame that you—and your inner child—carry from being abused, criticized, or ignored.

- Self-loathing for eating triggers the self-loathing that you—and your inner child—carry from believing you're unworthy of love and acceptance.

The situations may seem unrelated, but on a feeling level, they're linked. If these painful trauma-based emotions weren't already living in your mind and body, you wouldn't experience them so intensely just for eating a pizza. Beating yourself up for emotionally eating (it's not a sin!) keeps you experiencing these feelings over and over again and makes it harder to heal from early trauma and emotional eating.

You can disrupt and weaken this link—and eventually heal emotional eating—by ending an overeating episode with tenderness instead of punishment, with love instead of hate.

This is your key to success.

Notice what happens when you speak to yourself with tenderness after eating a tub of ice cream. Instead of berating yourself, you say: "I was lonely last night and overdid it with the ice cream. It's okay. In time, I'll use other ways to soothe my feelings."

Self-compassion feels better, doesn't it? It not only gives you present-day relief, but it also offers healing to the unprocessed pain inside of you.

Remember this: the times you treat yourself with tenderness and love after emotionally eating are more important signs of progress—of healing emotional eating *and* childhood abuse and trauma—than times you don't emotionally eat.

Speak to Yourself with Compassion

Upon entering my office, Teresa looked tired. Her strained smile and droopy eyes conveyed sadness. "I didn't want to come today," she said.

Knowing this meant Teresa was reluctant to discuss something, I said, "Okay...what is it you don't want to talk about?"

Teresa took a deep breath and said, "I had a bad day at work yesterday. I made a mistake, and my boss got mad at me. I was so ashamed that last night I ate an entire box of chocolate chip cookies. I was angry with myself for doing that, and then I couldn't fall asleep. I'm exhausted."

After a moment of silence, I said, "Teresa, it's okay. Really."

"I don't want to keep eating like that, but I can't seem to stop. I feel like a loser," she said.

"You can be so hard on yourself," I said. "Let's look at this another way."

I asked Teresa how her mother, a single, overwhelmed, and depressed woman, disciplined her when she was a child. Clutching her long bead necklace she said, "She hit me, yelled all the time, and called me stupid." Teresa had been a quiet, shy child, but her emotionally immature mother abused and lashed out at her simply for being a kid. In her mother's eyes, nothing Teresa did was right.

"What did you need back then, Teresa?" I asked. She became quiet and then said, "I guess I needed someone to tell me I was a good girl."

"Yes...you did need that, Teresa," I said. "Can you see how you're treating yourself the same way your mother treated you? When you beat yourself up for eating or for the mistake you made at work—eating cookies is not a big deal, and we all make mistakes—you're abusing yourself the way *she* abused you. That precious little girl inside of you keeps getting hurt, over and over again."

Teresa's eyes got misty. We had spoken about this before, but now it resonated more deeply. She said, "I'm treating myself so badly, aren't I?"

"Yes, you are," I said. "And that's understandable. It's what you learned. But you have to stop doing that to yourself. It's hurting you. And it's hurting that little girl inside you too. Abusing yourself for eating cookies and making a mistake adds to your pain. I promise you, treating yourself with kindness and love—instead of hate—will help. And it will help heal the part of you that believes you deserve to be abused."

Teresa understood and opened to a new way of talking to herself after emotionally eating. I explained that the self-punishing voices in her head would continue, but with patience and persistence, she could quiet them. We discussed how she could use compassionate self-talk after emotionally eating to support and reassure herself. Here are some phrases that felt authentic and true for Teresa. How do they sound to you?

- "Eating the _____ is *not* a big deal. I will put it in perspective and let it go."

- "It's okay. Habits take time to change. I'm doing the best I can."

- "I love and accept myself no matter what. Overeating doesn't define who I am."

- "No way I'll let this ruin my day. Onward!"

Once Teresa understood that berating herself for emotionally eating was self-abuse—and repeated the trauma she experienced as a child—she began to make huge strides. It took time to become more self-loving, but little by little, she succeeded. In particular, three things changed for her:

1. As she committed to being less harsh and angry with herself, she felt less judgmental and angry toward others. This lessened the frequency of anger-induced emotional eating.

2. While she continued to use food to cope at times, it became easier to use other ways to comfort herself and calm her body when triggered. After a while, these other ways—wearing her sacred shawl, writing in her journal, knitting—became routine self-care habits.

3. She felt greater compassion for herself, and this transferred to her body too. It felt easier to give her body movement, and she looked forward to taking her body on "walking dates."

Ending self-punishment for emotional eating helped Teresa stop perpetuating the pain from childhood abuse and trauma, and this was crucial to helping her heal. As she released this weight from her heart, emotional eating triggers lessened too.

My suggestion to you, like with Teresa, is to begin developing habits of self-compassion and tender emotional self-care, especially when trauma-based shame, guilt, and self-loathing emerge after eating. To start, use Teresa's self-talk statements above. Use the phrases that feel natural to you and feel free to add new ones. Write these down in your journal to affirm the new beliefs you're creating and have them available when you need them.

Remember, your goal right now isn't to stop emotionally eating. It's to give yourself love and tenderness when you do.

Despite your best intentions, you will emotionally eat. At these times, your trauma-based crew of fears and limiting beliefs will sow seeds of doubt in your mind and try to sabotage you. They want to prove to you that you cannot stop emotionally eating. They will taunt you with thoughts like these:

"See? Nothing works."

"I've tried everything and fail each time."

"It's hopeless. I can't do this."

Sound familiar?

These self-defeating thoughts will try to hijack your mind. Recognize them for the lies they are and use them to *strengthen* rather than weaken you. Each time you hear them, say, "Hello. Here you are again. Thank you for reminding me to be kind to myself. Bye-bye now." And remember to add love to your sacred vessel when your crew of fears cries out.

Harnessing confident, compassionate self-talk may not eliminate these sabotaging thoughts and lies from your mind right away. They're pesky and rooted in fear, and they will return. That's okay. It's how you respond to them, each and every time, that helps reduce their power over you. Be persistent.

In the same way you needed an adult to stop the hurt and soothe your pain, be your own best parent. Even if you didn't experience reassurance when you were a child, you can use reassuring words to comfort yourself today. Eventually, a gentle, reassuring voice will soon take root in your mind.

Think of Yourself in a New Way

My clients often say, "If I stop turning to food when I'm upset, what will I do? Food has been like my best friend. I'll feel lost." Or they say, "My problem is I just love food. I don't want to give up that pleasure."

Can you relate?

When you fear you're losing something you've relied on to cope, it feels destabilizing. Until you learn new habits, old ones serve a purpose. And, of course, you never have to give up the pleasure of your favorite foods. My suggestion to clients—and to you—is this: instead of asking yourself what you will do if you stop using food to cope, ask: "Who do I become?"

This question helps you move from fear to trust. Take a moment, get quiet, and ask yourself (or your Wise Self) this question. Notice what you hear. If you don't hear anything right now, that's okay. If you do, write it down in your journal.

Your self-perception—what you believe to be true about yourself—guides your behavior. Asking and journaling on "Who do I become?" helps you bypass fear and expand your mind to a new way of seeing yourself. Instead of giving attention to fears that challenge your healing, you focus *on the person you're becoming in the process*. This helps you create not just the possibility but the *probability* of your new normal. A new normal that is fueled by faith instead of hijacked by fear. After journaling on this question, Teresa wrote:

"When I stop relying on food to cope—and stop beating myself up when I do—I become someone who can comfort herself the way my mother couldn't. I use loving ways to soothe myself. I no longer mindlessly eat. I give myself nutritious food in satisfying portions. I accept my feelings—even the hard ones. I'm kind to myself."

What about you? What new possibilities open up when you reflect on the person you're becoming? If you'd like, write in your journal using this prompt: "When I no longer use food to cope—and stop beating myself up when I do—I become someone who..."

Mental Rehearsal: Envisioning the New You

Now let's take it a step further with a visualization exercise called mental rehearsal. When we imagine and rehearse in our mind new ways of seeing ourselves, we're rewiring our brain to create a new roadmap for the future. Sport psychologists teach elite athletes how to use visualization along with physical training. They practice and rehearse skills with their bodies *and* with their minds. But you don't need to be an Olympic gold medalist to benefit from the power of visualization. This exercise will help you practice and internalize using self-compassion after emotionally eating. Here's what you do:

1. Start by thinking about a time you were triggered, used food to cope, and then berated yourself. This will be the image you use to mentally rehearse using self-compassion.

2. Then, get yourself comfortable, sitting or lying down, in a quiet space with no distractions. Breathe diaphragmatically to calm and settle your mind and body. Close your eyes.

3. Now, as if you're the director of a movie, you'll recreate that scene in your mind. Do your best to capture all the senses: what you see, hear, smell, taste, and feel. Most people are attuned to certain senses more than others, so no worries if it's not all clear to you. Just imagine to the best of your ability. The more you do this, the easier it becomes.

4. Imagine yourself in this experience starting from when you got triggered through emotionally eating. But this time, instead of beating yourself up afterward, imagine using self-compassion. For example, visualize the situation that triggered you and how you then used food to cope. Then, imagine getting your sacred shawl and hugging yourself saying, "It's okay. Eating that cake was not a big deal. I won't let it ruin my day." Then, visualize yourself reading a book of daily meditations for further upliftment and peace.

5. Stay with the soothing ending of this image for several minutes or as long as feels comfortable. When done, allow the scene to fade from your mind and then open your eyes. Write about the experience in your journal. What does the new ending look like? How does it feel to use self-love instead of hate?

6. Use visualization to plant seeds of growth in your mind and brain and imagine yourself as the self-compassionate person you're becoming. Practice using this exercise with different emotional eating experiences and create your new ending. The mind doesn't know the difference between what's real and what you imagine, so when you mentally rehearse new behaviors, your mind internalizes them as if they are real. This helps rewire your brain to support these new choices.

As you visualize yourself "being" the person you want to become—a self-compassionate person who enjoys a peaceful relationship with food, feelings, and your body—you set in motion neurological and unconscious forces to help you move in that direction because your brain begins to think that the future *is today*. (You'll find one of my favorite guided imagery books in the "Resources" section.)

Staying Focused, Calm, and Comforted

Planning ahead helps you take charge of emotional eating and its aftermath so it stops taking charge of you. As you become a more powerful person who no longer needs food to cope, here's a gift I'd like you to create for yourself—and your inner child: a love note for support and guidance.

By writing your love note now, you can read it when you need support after an emotional eating episode. Here's what you do:

1. Give yourself about thirty minutes of quiet time with no distractions. Thinking about yourself as your own best friend, write yourself a note of reassurance and support. What would a best friend say when you're berating yourself? What would *you* say to a best friend struggling with emotional eating? Or imagine that your Wise Self is writing to you. What would she say? What words do you need to hear when you're overwhelmed and upset? What words did the child you once were need to hear when they were overwhelmed and upset? (You can listen to the Wise Self audio that offers guidance to use in your note, which is available at http://www.newharbinger. com/51178.)

2. Start your note with *Dear* _____ and add your name. Does your best friend or Wise Self call you "Darling" or "Sweetie"? If so, address yourself that way.

3. As you write, offer yourself praise for committing to take good care of yourself. Tell yourself you are valued and precious. Offer yourself acceptance for times you emotionally eat along with reassurance that you are growing and healing. Encourage yourself to be patient.

4. Include reminders to use specific strategies you've learned for soothing and self-compassion. For example, you could mention items from your self-care basket. Write in your note whatever you believe that you—and your inner child—need to hear for reassurance and support after emotionally eating. Here's Teresa's note from her Wise Self.

Darling Teresa,

You deserve to be cherished. Don't be so hard on yourself, dear. You're doing a great job committing to your well-being. Be gentle and patient with yourself.

I think you need a hug. If you're able, wear your sacred shawl and hug yourself. Imagine I'm hugging you too. I'm right here. Can you feel me? You're not alone, darling.

Breathe for a few minutes to settle yourself. Just allow the feelings to wash through your body. It's okay. Your feelings can't hurt you. Perhaps you'd like to use progressive muscle relaxation on your arms and legs to ground and settle yourself further.

Emotional eating is not a sin, remember? You're doing the best you can. Using food for comfort is a habit you learned, and you're taking steps to change that. The most important thing right now is to be kind to yourself. You can later discuss with a friend or write in your journal about what triggered the urge to eat. This will help you process what happened without food getting in the way.

Perhaps you'd like to get your knitting project from your self-care basket and work on that for ten minutes. Or find something else from your basket that will help you feel soothed.

Hold faith in your heart, darling. You're growing wiser and stronger every day. You've got this.

Love,

Your Wise Self

Write your note on plain paper first. That way, you don't need to worry about penmanship or getting it right. When you're done, you can rewrite it on special paper or a pretty note card. Keep your note with you all the time. You may want to make two or three copies and keep them in different places, such as your purse, bedside table, and kitchen drawer.

Read your note after you emotionally eat—because you will, *and that's okay.* Read slowly and thoughtfully. Feel your note's loving energy fill your mind, body, and spirit. You'll find comfort in knowing that encouragement and support—and hearing your Wise Self's loving words—are only a piece of paper away.

Putting It All Together

When you have a history of trauma and struggle with emotional eating, it sometimes feels impossible to cope without the quick fix of food. In this chapter, you learned that creating gentler, compassionate self-talk *after* emotionally eating is ultimately more important than whether or not you stop using food to cope right now. This is the key to your success and paves the way for sustained healing—for emotional eating *and* early trauma.

Practicing the self-talk, writing, and imagery exercises you learned in this chapter, along with reading your love note, will help you create and reinforce loving ways of seeing and caring for yourself. These self-compassion practices help you begin to naturally give yourself love and support. And this changes and heals *everything.*

In the next chapter, you'll learn a different approach and how changing your *outer* environment helps you create inner change too.

CHAPTER 9

Create an Emotionally Safe Sanctuary

In previous chapters, you learned about healing childhood trauma and emotional eating by calming your nervous system, improving your relationship with your body, releasing subconscious beliefs, processing feelings, making peace with trigger foods, and harnessing the power of self-compassion. These approaches help you heal from the *inside out*. When you change *internal* physiological states, beliefs, and feelings, you create *external* change with the empowered choices that these inner shifts help you make. In this chapter, you'll learn a different approach. Not often associated with psychological healing and self-growth, clutter clearing helps you create life-transforming change from the *outside in*.

I learned about the power of clutter clearing to create an emotionally safe home environment from space clearing expert Karen Kingston (1998), author of *Clear Your Clutter with Feng Shui: Free Yourself From Physical, Mental, Emotional, and Spiritual Clutter Forever*. This book transformed my life. So they could benefit too, I began teaching this process to my clients. I consider it emotional growth's best-kept secret.

Kingston teaches about the energetic impact of clutter on your physical, emotional, and spiritual health. Especially for people who experienced childhood trauma and keep objects from their past, this information is invaluable. I won't be addressing the impact of general household clutter, although that's important. What you'll learn in this chapter is the power of releasing items that hold the symbolism and energy of trauma, which keep you anchored in the past, and how to be discerning with objects and symbols you bring into your life today.

As you learned in chapter 5, to heal emotional eating and childhood trauma, your conscious and subconscious minds must agree with the plan. Releasing physical objects that hold the energy of painful experiences is another way to align your two minds so they'll stop competing with each other and allow your healing journey to flow more smoothly. This is like opening the lid to your subconscious container and removing fears and limiting beliefs.

Everything is energy, and we hold energy in different ways: in the cells of our body; in our thoughts, feelings, and conscious and subconscious beliefs; in the tangible objects we own; and in the unseen space radiating out from our physical body, which is referred to as our energy field. We are attached to our living space and personal belongings—home, vehicle, purse—by invisible threads of energy flowing around and through us. You can't see them, but they affect you nevertheless because everything you own is embedded with and reinforces the energy of your beliefs. This is how objects from a traumatic childhood can hold you hostage to your past. The concrete, visible world of our "stuff" and the invisible world of our emotions and energy field are one. It's all connected.

When you release objects from your outside world that no longer serve you, you energetically release what no longer serves you *on the inside* as well. For example, by letting go of outdated clothes from an earlier—and perhaps, harder—time in your life, you begin to let go of outdated beliefs about yourself too. You essentially release the energy held in those pieces of clothing—from the outside *and* inside of you. In this chapter, I will teach you how to look at your home and belongings with new eyes and how taking concrete steps can help clean your energy field and, subsequently, strengthen your self-worth.

Releasing what no longer supports you and your life is an act of radical self-respect. It can feel hard to let go of our belongings, especially sentimental items. But removing things that remind you of people, places, and events that hold pain from the past helps open space for new joyful experiences. Have you heard the saying "nature abhors a vacuum"? What that means is as you create space by releasing objects and symbols that hold the energy of trauma and emotional eating struggles, energetic forces naturally fill that space to support the new person you're becoming. This doesn't necessarily mean the space refills with more "stuff." Energetically, these newly opened spaces help create more joyful *internal* states. This is how targeted clutter clearing helps you release the old so you can make way for the *new you*.

Our homes and belongings are like mirrors reflecting to us the beliefs we hold of ourselves. As you look around your environment, what do you see? Do you see objects that uplift your spirit or drain you? Are you reminded of loving memories or painful ones? Sometimes we're so used to having items in our lives that we don't "see" their deeper meaning or "feel" the effect on our spirit. This doesn't mean you let go of everything from your childhood, although you may choose to. It means you look critically at what you own, release items associated with painful experiences, and keep only those items that bring joy and comfort to your heart.

The information and examples in this chapter will help expand how you view your belongings so you can make mindful choices about what to keep and what to release. We'll start with the following list, which includes items some of my clients discovered were associated with disappointment, sadness, and fear. Notice how you feel as you read and if your mind wanders to things you own that resonate with this list. If you wish, read this list (and chapter) while wearing your sacred shawl so your Wise Self can offer comfort if needed.

- Diaries filled with loneliness, sadness, despair.

- The teddy bear, baby doll, or blanket you hugged while crying yourself to sleep.

- Pictures of family members with angry or sad facial expressions.

- Photos of the person or people who abused you. (It may feel easier to discard photos of people with whom you did not feel emotionally attached. However, when the person who abused you also is someone you loved, it may feel more complicated. In this case, you may want to keep some photos, but consider releasing those that feel unsettling to you for any reason.)

- Favorite books you read or games you played to help you emotionally escape.

- The gold bracelet your grandfather gave you on your thirteenth birthday. You knew this was his way of bribing you to "keep our secret" about sexually abusing you.

- The Christmas tree angel that witnessed holiday arguments and fights.

- Dishware that may be useful but holds the energy of mealtime family tension.

- The vintage radio with a crack from when your father threw it against the wall.

- School papers, books, or report cards from those years of wondering how you'll ever get through another day.

Let's pause here. How are you doing? Even if the examples do not exactly apply to you, they may trigger sorrow. Take a break if you need to. Hug yourself with your sacred shawl. Perhaps you'd like to write in your journal to process memories that may be emerging. Come back when you're ready.

I'll now share three examples to help you learn how releasing trauma-related items can support your healing journey.

Susan's Piggy Bank

Susan entered therapy to heal emotional eating, which began during her lonely and emotionally neglectful childhood. After she made some progress, I introduced the concept of clutter clearing to help her heal "from the outside in." Susan told me about a jewelry box with a twirling ballerina on its lid that her mother gave her when she was four years old. She keeps it on her bedroom bureau. When she looks at the jewelry box, it puts a smile on her face.

Susan also kept a metal piggy bank next to the jewelry box. This was a gift from her maternal grandfather, Papa, for her tenth birthday. Papa was a mean-spirited, wealthy man whom Susan feared and who died when she was twenty-five. While he never hurt Susan, he physically abused Susan's mother when she was growing up. When Susan learned this, it helped her understand why her mother was chronically depressed and emotionally unavailable. Susan knew her grandfather used his money in manipulative ways yet was stunned to learn that he cut Susan's mother out of his will.

After learning about the power of clutter clearing, Susan kept the jewelry box that gave her much joy but decided to get rid of the piggy bank. She said, "It felt liberating because I respected myself enough to take a stand against injustice. I have compassion for my grandfather because he was abused as a child too. But keeping the piggy bank with its money symbolism no longer felt right. I don't want the energy of abuse and vindictiveness in my home anymore."

Beth's Kitty

As a child and teen, Beth loved her stuffed animals. Of all the ones that slept on her bed every night, only beloved Kitty joined Beth's journey into adulthood. Her paternal grandmother, Nana, gave this to Beth when she was five years old.

Beth worked hard in therapy to heal from growing up with parents who abused drugs and neglected her emotional, physical, and medical needs. The only love Beth experienced as a child was from Nana. Clutching Kitty at night helped Beth endure a sad and lonely childhood.

Beth's first recollection of binge eating was when she was eight years old. Nana had just died, and she recalled eating donuts at the funeral. "I was overcome with grief, but no one asked me how I felt. I kept going back for more donuts. I think they distracted me from the hole I felt in my heart. After Nana died, I felt lost." Beth discovered that food—not people— soothed her painful feelings. Donuts, cookies, and sweets, along with Kitty, became trusted companions.

As Beth healed from the trauma she experienced, her confidence, inner security, and self-worth improved. While she no longer fell asleep hugging Kitty at night, she still kept her on a chair in her bedroom.

I had discussed with Beth the power of clutter cleaning, and during our work together, she discarded many objects from her childhood. In one session, I asked if she still needed Kitty in her life. My question prompted Beth to look at Kitty differently. She took time to decide what to do with this beloved stuffed animal that provided much comfort when she was a child.

Several sessions later, Beth said, "I think I'm ready to let go of Kitty. She was my constant companion through hard times in my life, but I'm not there anymore. And while Kitty reminds me of my grandmother's love, she also reminds me of how I *didn't* feel loved by my parents. I feel my grand- mother's love all the time. I don't want to be reminded of the pain anymore."

Beth wasn't sure how to let go of Kitty. She didn't want to put her in the trash, and Kitty was too worn out to be donated. I suggested that Beth give Kitty a proper burial. She loved the idea and created a ritual. Beth wrote two letters: one to Nana, thanking her for being so loving, and the other to Kitty, thanking her for giving her comfort during those painful years. She dug a hole in her yard, buried Kitty with the letters, and planted a rose bush.

When Beth looks at the rosebush, she feels peace. Kitty (and food) offered Beth the only comfort she knew at a time she felt vulnerable and alone. "Since removing Kitty from my bedroom and burying her," Beth said, "I feel lighter. I'm not a child who needs that kind of security anymore. I think this helps with not impulsively grabbing food so much too. I feel stronger." (If you have a stuffed animal or blanket from childhood that continues to give you comfort, I'm not suggesting you discard it. That was Beth's choice. You choose what's best for you.)

Jenna's Diaries

When Jenna started therapy, she was depressed and struggled with C-PTSD symptoms from years of emotional and physical abuse by her step-father and older brothers. Anxiety-filled days and lonely nights often ended with Jenna eating herself into a food coma.

As a child, Jenna discovered that food numbed her pain. She learned that writing helped too. Jenna's aunt had given her a diary when she was ten years old. Through years of silently enduring abuse, Jenna found comfort in writing. She wrote about girlfriend gossip, the stress of home-work, and how much she hated her life.

As a sensitive thirty-seven-year-old woman, Jenna made great strides in therapy. She began to feel less depressed, more hopeful about her future, and emotional eating lessened. It took time, but Jenna began to love and value herself for the first time in her life.

When we discussed the power of clutter clearing to turn her home into an emotionally safe sanctuary, Jenna immediately got on board. She got rid of clothes, books, kitchenware—anything she no longer found useful or reminded her of painful times in her life.

Jenna had saved her childhood diaries and the journals she wrote in as an adult. As she embraced the power of clutter clearing, she knew she had to do something with them. She said, "From everything I've learned about clutter clearing, I know these diaries have to go. They're filled with so much pain. Writing has been my lifesaver, but it's time to get the pain on those pages out of my life."

Jenna created a letting-go ritual to release her diaries. The process took several days. She lived in an apartment with a fireplace, so she gathered her diaries and put them in her living room. (If you're unable to burn paper items safely, you can shred them.) Sitting cross-legged on the floor, Jenna skimmed through the entries in each diary and journal. She thanked them for helping her through her tough childhood. She then burned them in the fireplace. She said, "It felt freeing to let them go. I felt sad at times reading the entries—sad for the little girl I was and for how lonely I've felt as an adult—but also lighter. Right afterward, I felt the impulse to go for a walk. My body felt energized. I've done a lot of work to heal, and this was exactly what I needed to do to bring myself to the next level."

Clutter clearing sometimes can produce rapid, profound results. Two months after burning her diaries, which also included entries about the pain of numerous failed relationships, Jenna met the love of her life while walking her dog. It wasn't only releasing the diaries that helped Jenna find a fulfilling relationship. She had worked hard by using the inside-out processes in this book and made great progress. But releasing the diaries energetically helped Jenna open to joy and move her life to the next level.

There are different ways to release objects you own that hold cobwebs of sadness and pain. Some people discard or donate them, like Susan did with the piggy bank. Others, like Jenna and Beth, find comfort in performing a release or burial ritual. It's your *intention* behind releasing the object that's important. These are examples. Use them as inspiration to find what works best for you.

New Arrivals

Now let's talk about items you acquired as an adult. The objects and symbols surrounding you tell a story about your life. As you read the three examples below, reflect on your own belongings and notice if any may be rooted in trauma, abuse, and emotional eating challenges. Let's look at Jerry's life and the story his objects were telling.

Jerry entered therapy due to severe anxiety and depression. A perceptive, quick-witted man, he didn't realize how being physically abused by his father had affected his life. His way of coping with overwhelming emotion was to drink beer and eat. Jerry wore a black leather jacket with a skull and crossbones painted across the back, and coupled with the metal bullet dangling from his right ear, his appearance conveyed an aura of toughness. As I got to know Jerry, I learned how gentle and sensitive he is. In one session, I asked him why he had a bullet as an earring. He said, "I don't know. I just like it." I explained that sometimes the symbols in our life tell a story, and I wondered what story that bullet and the skull and crossbones were telling. I said, "You're such a kind and gentle person. These symbols don't fit who you are. Who do they really belong to?"

My question triggered a memory of Jerry's father threatening his mother with a gun and Jerry trying to protect her. "My father was a mean bastard," he said. "It was okay that he beat me, but I had to stand up to him or I feared that he'd kill my mother. As we're talking about this, I'm thinking that the jacket and bullet help me feel tough so that people won't take advantage of me. Wow—I never realized this meant anything, but I see what you're saying. I'm wearing this earring to try to protect the boy I was."

Not long after that session, Jerry removed the bullet earring. He kept the jacket for a while but later bought a plain one. He said, "As we've been working together around my father's violence, I've become a more confident person. I don't need to project that tough image anymore." Jerry had developed the confidence to release these symbols, and in turn, releasing these symbols strengthened his confidence.

Now let's look at Kristen's life and the story one of her shirts was telling.

Sexually abused by her stepfather from the age of eight until age sixteen, Kristen started therapy for help with chronic anxiety and emotional eating. She was making good progress. One day, she came to a session wearing blue jeans and a pink T-shirt with a white Playboy logo. After a moment I said, "Kristen, what does that shirt mean to you?" "Huh?" she said, "What do you mean?" "Well," I said, "it has a Playboy logo on it, and I wonder what it means for you to wear something that symbolizes sex." Kristen stared at me. After a moment she said, "I never thought of it like that. I just thought the pink and white looked pretty. But as soon as you said it symbolizes sex, my stepfather came to mind. I always felt like I was his whore, and he was cheating on my mother with me."

We discussed the T-shirt and the story Kristen's subconscious mind was still telling. Her eyes welled with tears. "Look what I'm doing to myself. It's like a part of me still feels dirty. I remember stuffing myself with cookies after my stepfather would leave my bedroom. I thought I was a horrible kid for betraying my mother."

"It's okay, Kristen," I said. "I know you believed that when you were a little girl. And it's not true. Let's take this is as an opportunity to reassure her—and you—that she's a good little girl who was terribly hurt." After Kristen and I discussed what it meant to keep or discard the T-shirt, she said, "When I get home, I'm throwing this away. Little Kristen has spent too many years feeling ashamed of herself, and I've reinforced that by wearing this. I'm not going to do that anymore."

When Kristen bought the T-shirt, she was oblivious to its meaning. As she said, she liked the colors. She truly didn't "see" the significance of wearing a logo that symbolized sex. The inner shame of feeling like a "whore" subconsciously compelled Kristen to buy the T-shirt. Hidden in plain sight, Kristen's outer world displayed what her inner world believed.

When the light of awareness shined on Kristen's choice to buy and wear that T-shirt, she could make a mindful decision about whether or not she wanted to keep it. Deciding to throw it away was an act of radical self-respect that removed those shame-based energies from Kristen's life. This fostered change from the "outside in" as she embraced a new and more respectful self-concept.

In our society, the lines can get blurry when it comes to sexual issues. Wearing a Playboy T-shirt, sharing silly sexual memes on social media, or telling off-color jokes may not seem like a big deal on the surface. But what about the deeper meaning for some people? What about the deeper meaning for you? If you were sexually abused, notice the symbols around you that may reflect sexual disrespect. For example, figurines of a naked man or woman (I don't mean respectful art; I mean those silly objects you find in souvenir-type shops) or sexually suggestive images on clothing, key chains, or coffee mugs. On the surface, some of these items may seem innocent. But they're not. They represent a lack of respect for women and, with some items, for men too.

Thus far we've been looking at the symbolic meaning of objects, writings, and clothing. But it's not only about these tangible items. It's also important to be mindful about what you share on social media, the conversations you have with people, and the "jokes" you tell.

Let's look at how an "innocent" cartoon undermined Darla's healing from emotional eating.

Darla struggled with food and eating and regularly joked about it. She would say things like, "Chocolate calls out my name!" and "I'll have cake; it's somebody's birthday somewhere!" (Do you say things like this too?) As a psychotherapist, I hear the painful stories hiding behind the attempt at humor. Our culture is so inundated with this stuff—think about similar memes on your Facebook or Instagram feed—that we're desensitized to how unhelpful they can be.

Darla told me about a cartoon she kept on her refrigerator. The caption said, "Pie Calling." It was a picture of a woman clasping her hands over her ears to stop hearing the pie across the room yelling, *"Eat me…eat me!"*

This cartoon belittled Darla's emotional eating struggles, so I told her my thoughts. She dismissed it at first, but eventually understood. She said, "I never joke with my daughters about things that bother them. It's not right to do this to myself. And that's not the kind of role model I want to be for my girls."

Darla took a powerful stand against demeaning herself and threw away the cartoon. She said it felt liberating to no longer see her food struggles glaring at her face every day. It was an act of radical self-respect to remove a cartoon that seemed funny on the surface yet actually was a way she was being unkind to herself. When Darla looked at that cartoon—numerous times a day—it reminded her how food controlled her life. Sure, she could "joke" about it. But deep down, she knew it wasn't funny. That cartoon fed Darla's deeper fear that she *never* would break free from emotional eating. The pie would always win.

This isn't to suggest that there's anything "wrong" with pie. It's not about the pie. It's about Darla's struggles and how that cartoon belittled her very real challenges.

Kind-hearted joking in many situations is harmless. And humor certainly can ease a hard situation. But routinely joking about something that's important to you and has been a struggle *isn't* funny. It's disrespectful and being unkind to yourself. Your trauma and emotional eating journey have been challenging enough. You don't need to make it harder with cartoons and jokes that mock your struggles.

Remember: the objects surrounding you tell a story about your life and show you how you see yourself. What story are you and your objects telling?

JOURNAL PROMPTS

Write down the thoughts and feelings that emerged for you thus far while reading this chapter. Then, write your responses to the following prompts in your journal:

- When I look at objects from my childhood, I feel...

- Some things remind me of happy times, but others (identify which ones) remind me of...

- When I look at newer objects and clothing, I see a story about someone who is...

Practicing Radical Self-Respect

As you've been learning, negative energies embedded in your belongings and words—even if they're "jokes"—hurt you and make your healing journey harder. These energies filter into your mind, feeding you images of defeat and disrespect. And keeping old or new items that carry the energy of painful childhood experiences hold you hostage to your past. But when you look at your belongings, words, and social media through the eyes of *radical self-respect* and release what sabotages you and your healing, you create empowered change *from the outside in*.

Here are some suggestions to help you get started:

- Commit to stop joking about your struggles with food or your body. When others are joking or complaining about these issues, choose not to participate. Offer a compassionate smile, be silent, or change the subject. Consider letting your friends know that you'll no longer belittle your challenges in this way. This doesn't mean you stop talking with them about your feelings. It means you engage them for emotional support and leave out the self-disrespect.

- When you see memes on social media that are supposed to be funny but really are sexually disrespectful, mean-spirited, fat-shaming, mental health shaming, aggressive, or mock your emotional eating challenges, don't share, "like," or comment. Unsubscribe from anything that contributes to hurting *anyone* so these posts no longer contaminate your media feeds—and your energy field.

- Look through your clothes and notice symbols that in any way promote harmful or sexually disrespectful or aggressive messages. If so, like Jerry and Kristen, consider getting rid of them.

- Look around your home, workspace, car, and purse. Notice what words and quotes you bring into your world via posters, kitchenware, and clothing. Get rid of anything that symbolizes trauma, abuse, despair, or in any way undermines your confidence and self-worth. For example, people who have struggled with relationships and feel emotionally isolated may be drawn to pictures of solitary people or animals. If this applies to you, consider shifting that energy and replace them with images that symbolize human connection. If you're not sure about the meaning your items convey, ask a friend who will tell you the truth.

- Whenever you buy something new, be discerning about the symbolic message you're bringing into your home and life. Go for images that evoke a light, confident, and joyous feeling compatible with the *new you*.

Putting It All Together

A holistic approach to healing includes *both inside-out and outside-in* approaches. It's important to practice techniques to calm your nervous system, soothe your feelings, shift your mindset from disempowering beliefs to empowering ones, and develop self-compassion. These *inside-out* strategies help you make sustained change. The additional support of *outside-in* strategies reinforces the inner changes you're making and accelerates your healing process. That's because the unseen world of energy holds immense power. This power can either hinder or help your healing. The suggestions you've learned in this chapter help you harness this power to support your progress. As you create changes in your external world, your internal world will change, too.

How about starting this week? Devote time to review items in one drawer, closet, or room. Reflect on the possible deeper meaning of some items. Write in your journal about what you noticed. Then, on another day, review items in a second drawer, closet, or room. Keep taking these small steps. You don't need to get rid of things immediately. The important thing right now is to examine your belongings and look at them through the lens of outside-in healing and radical self-respect. You then can develop a plan to throw things away, donate them, or create a clearing-out ritual. Once you get started, decluttering takes on a life of its own and can feel inspiring and freeing. So, lighten your load and begin healing *from the outside-in.*

We're nearing the end of our journey together. In the next section, we'll review where you've been, what you've learned, and what your future holds.

Parting Words

Congratulations for reading all the way through. I'm proud of you and hope you're proud of you too. Some of the material wasn't easy and may have felt triggering. It takes courage to persevere, so praise yourself for entering those hard places. This book also offers you hope and inspiration. You've learned about the connection between early trauma and emotional eating and now understand that your struggles with food are not due to personal failing. Trauma causes inner chaos, and you've coped the best way you could. You now have a roadmap and effective strategies to help you move through that chaos and heal.

Healing is an ongoing process, and there is no quick cure. It took you a long time to get here and will take time to move through. And that's okay! This book is a starting place from where you were when you began reading. Remember: your Wise Self knows that *you have what it takes to heal* or you wouldn't have been drawn to this book in the first place.

In the "Welcome" and first two chapters, you learned foundational information including: how early trauma affects the brain and creates body dysregulation, how food offers an easy source of comfort, the importance of releasing traumatic secrets, the differences between emotional and physical hunger, and how to identify your body's hunger-fullness level. You also learned diaphragmatic breathing and progressive muscle relaxation, two self-calming strategies that require only your breath and body. Chapters 3 through 8 addressed specific topics, and you learned *inside-out* strategies to calm your nervous system, to create a respectful partnership with your body, to soothe and release subconscious fear-based thoughts, to mindfully process your feelings, to make peace with trigger foods, and how self-compassion is key to heal emotional eating. In chapter 9, you learned how to create an emotionally and energetically safe home sanctuary with an *out-side-in* healing approach of releasing trauma-based objects and symbols.

It's a lot of information, so take time to absorb it all.

If you haven't already, I encourage you to create your sacred shawl, sacred vessel, and self-care basket. They're useful and practical grounding tools, and once you have them, they're always there when needed. And remember to download your free audios—Meet Your Wise Self, Peaceful Place, Progressive Muscle Relaxation, Connect with Your Body-Wisdom— as well as the PDFs to gauge how safe your body feels, your hunger-fullness levels, and tools to process your feelings, along with the audio instruction guide, all available at http://www.newharbinger.com/51178.

Healing from trauma and emotional eating requires a willingness to make your emotional, physical, and spiritual self-care a priority; explore your inner world; and incorporate new practices into your daily life. By purchasing and reading this book, you've already shown that willingness. Good for you.

In my professional experience, the difference between people who move forward in their healing journey and get the results they want and those who have a harder time isn't based on knowledge and strategies alone, although that's important. People who are successful possess the following five qualities. Do you? If not, know that you can and imagine right now how much easier your healing journey will be as you develop them.

1. Patience

You need time to emotionally grow into the person you're becoming. Healing is a process, and patience gives your self-concept the time it needs to expand and grow beyond where you started. If change were to happen too quickly (and it doesn't), it would be too overwhelming to adjust to those shifts.

There will be days you feel frustrated and demoralized that change isn't happening fast enough, and you'll wonder, *What's the point?* When that happens, say to yourself: "I am the point." Then, hold faith in your heart, stay committed to *you*, and have patience.

2. Commitment to Consistent Practice

Devote time to take daily steps in the service of your healing and self-growth. For example, perhaps you listen to the progressive muscle relaxation audio to calm your nervous system, take one item from your self-care basket and give yourself "me" time not because you're triggered but because you deserve it, or as you learned in chapter 4, begin your day by asking your body, "What do you need from me today so you will feel loved and well-cared for?"

People get better long-term results by doing small things every single day, with one caveat. Every day doesn't mean you won't miss a day. Or two. Or three. Life happens. Every day means *every day that you can.* When you miss some days, start anew the next day with commitment sans guilt.

3. Self-Compassion

Self-compassion is a soothing balm that transforms suffering into healing. That's why it's important to give yourself love and tenderness. It's what helps you heal and grow. The negative words you say to yourself are your worst enemies, while words of self-compassion are your greatest friends. So instead of beating yourself up with harsh words, *lift yourself up* with kindness. (When you feel stuck in negativity after using food to cope, review "Transform Self-Punishment into Self-Compassion" in chapter 8.)

4. Self-Responsibility

Healing and self-growth happen more steadily when people take responsibility for themselves and their actions. They do not blame others, make excuses for their behavior, or relentlessly complain about their life. For example, they accept they used food when upset without blaming their partner for "making them angry." Taking responsibility for your feelings and actions—with love and self-compassion—helps you develop the confidence and integrity necessary for sustained healing.

5. Perseverance

Stick with your healing journey despite feeling discouraged. And you *will* feel discouraged at times. That's being human, and it's okay. Remember this: perseverance is trust in action. It means you take those small daily steps—and some large ones—even when you don't see the results you want but trust that you will over time. That steady willingness to persevere *is* progress.

Healing from trauma and emotional eating—healing from anything, really—does not follow a straight path. It has ups and downs and a forward-backward momentum. You'll have days when it feels easy to self-soothe without turning to food and days when you can't stop grabbing fistfuls of chips. You'll have days when you feel such deep pain that it's hard to get out of bed in the morning and days when your soul is filled with gratitude for the blessings in your life.

All change—including healing emotional eating and childhood trauma—is a process that goes something like this:

You take one or two steps forward, then one step back. Three steps forward and another step or two back. Then forward again. And so on. Backward steps are when you fall into old habits and responses. For example, feeling emotionally triggered when you thought you were *so over that,* using food to soothe yourself after you haven't for months, or not using self-care strategies when you need them.

What you may think is going backward is actually *growth in disguise.* When we open ourselves to growing and changing, it can trigger fear that pulls us back into old patterns. Revisiting these old patterns is necessary because each time they happen you're given the opportunity to use the tools you've learned and strengthen the habit of becoming your new you. Each time you take a forward-moving step—after a backward one—you strengthen your commitment, challenge limiting beliefs, and practice the new skills you're learning. That's how you make sustained progress. It's this consistent practice, especially when you feel discouraged, that helps you move forward. And practice is most effective when it's fueled with patience, self-responsibility, self-compassion, and perseverance.

Think about it: Babies don't just climb out of the crib and walk, right? They stand for a second, and then fall, without self-judgment—over and over and over again—as they develop balance, coordination, and confidence. And then they walk. Can you imagine if after the first few tries, we all had said, "This walking is too hard, I keep falling—I'm done." We'd all still be crawling around!

Within your healing journey, you will falter. You will fumble. You will fall too, just as you did when you were learning to walk.

And that's okay.

There's no set finish line to healing trauma and emotional eating, so I want you to look at it this way. Think of a continuum from 1 to 100. Perhaps right now when hard feelings surface, your emotions and body dysregulation are at 90 to 100 percent intensity, so you feel completely overwhelmed. You feel triggered to eat 90 to 100 percent of the time when that happens. Progress doesn't mean you'll never feel triggered and stop emotionally eating completely. This is what it means:

As you heal, painful emotional reactions occur less frequently, feel less intense, and last for shorter periods of time. For example, instead of feeling triggered with 90 to 100 percent intensity, you've worked at calming your nervous system and noticing, naming, accepting, and loving your feelings so that the intensity of feeling triggered moves down to 60, 40, or 30 percent. And instead of turning to food 90 to 100 percent of the time, you turn to food 60, 40, or 30 percent of the time. Healing emotional eating doesn't necessarily mean that you'll get to 0 percent of being triggered and stop emotionally eating completely. *And that's okay.* At some point, you'll get down to 10, 20, or 30 percent of frequency and intensity—and you can live successfully with that.

I want to remind you that you will meet some inner resistance along your healing journey. This is typical. As you learned in chapter 5, your subconscious beliefs will resist change and try to prove to you that "this isn't working." When that happens, speak to those thoughts and beliefs. For example, when you hear taunting voices in your head saying, "I'll never stop using food to cope," or "I'll always feel like a failure," or "This pain will never stop," say to those voices, "Thank you for reminding me to be kind to myself." Then, wrap yourself in your sacred shawl, add love to your sacred vessel, and stay committed to you.

One way to stay committed is to remind yourself of these four important words: *I have a choice.*

Every moment in every day we make choices. When you feel triggered to eat, you can choose to emotionally eat or soothe yourself in another way. If you choose to emotionally eat, afterward, you can choose to be cruel to yourself or kind. You have options. Lots of them really, and you've learned many in this book. But it's hard to see those options when trauma-filled thoughts and sensations hijack your mind and body and cloud your judgment, and you feel overwhelmed and stuck. And you *will* feel stuck sometimes because you're human and healing is never a straight line. So I'd like you to write these four words—*I Have a Choice*—on a card or in your phone to keep handy and read the next time you need a reminder that you're not helpless, it's not hopeless, and you're more in control of your actions than you may think.

Healing Is Possible

It's not easy to have a history of trauma and struggle with emotional eating at the same time, but I promise, healing will happen as you're ready. And I know that you're ready because here you are. I trust you know this too.

Healing the pain from your past transforms your life. You find strength by moving through your vulnerability, courage by facing your fears, and self-love through embracing the hurt little child inside you. As that happens, and by consistently using the tools you learned in this book—along with patience, commitment, self-responsibility, self-compassion, and perseverance—you free yourself for a life of contentment, emotional strength, and unconditional self-love.

Thank you for reading this book and allowing me to accompany you on your journey. I wish you peace and happiness.

With love,

Diane

Acknowledgments

This book began decades ago, before I wrote the first word. To my early supporters, thank you for helping me get started. To those who later joined my journey, I am grateful. I couldn't have done this without your help.

Heartfelt thanks to Mary Hartley, RD. You've traveled this path with me from day one. Thank you for your friendship, believing in me, your insights, and for reading portions of my manuscript. I am grateful to you.

Thank you to David Jacques, Elizabeth Sanberg, Cori Chong, and Alana Riley, for helping me bring my work out of my office and into the world. And to Hillary Sciscoe, thank you for keeping it going.

To Madeleine Eno, thank you for your amazing editing and content-building help in those early, and later, years. I learned so much from you.

Thank you to Donna Rustigian Mac for your audio direction and production, and for helping me make the beautiful recordings that accompany this book. It's been a pleasure to work with you over the years.

To Renee Brochester, MSW; Barbara Frame, MSW; and Kristen Harrington, MA. Thank you for reading portions of my manuscript and for your helpful feedback.

To Lisa Tener, thank you for your awesome book-coaching and teaching me about proposal-writing and publishing. Whenever I had a question, you were right there. Your help and support were invaluable.

To my writing mentor, Debra Landwehr Engle. You held my hand as I conceptualized and wrote the proposal and first draft of this book. Thank you for all the ways you helped me realize my dream. Deep gratitude to you.

Heartfelt thanks to Georgia Kolias, my book angel, and editor at New Harbinger Publications. It wasn't random. The Universe put my proposal in your hands for a reason. Thank you for being my champion. Your belief in me and my writing has been breathtaking. Grateful to you, always.

And thank you to my team at New Harbinger. To Madison Davis, Gretel Hakanson, Callie Brown, and Amy Shoup (for your beautiful cover design), it was a pleasure to work with you. And to all who helped bring this book into the world, I am grateful to you and for the opportunity New Harbinger has given me.

To Donna Jackson Nakazawa, thank you for taking time out of your busy schedule to write the foreword to this book. I am so grateful. And thank you for helping the world heal and thrive with your amazing books and teachings. We all are grateful.

To my dear friend, Cate McQuaid. Where do I begin? You held my hand and walked with me every step of the way. Your insightful feedback on my manuscript and loyal support kept me inspired and reassured. Your friendship warms my soul. Thank you so much. I am grateful for you.

To my former therapist, Leland DeVoli, DO. You helped save my emotional life. Grateful to you forever.

Deep gratitude to my spiritual teachers Sanaya Roman (channel for Orin), Paramahansa Yogananda, and Ihaleakala Hew Len, PhD, who taught me the healing practice of Ho'oponopono. Your teachings have inspired my life and my work. Thank you.

To my clients, thank you for sharing your lives with me and trusting me with your hearts. I am deeply honored.

To my father, Adelmo Petrella, who left too soon, and to my mother, Theresa Rossi Petrella, who gave me the gifts of love and time. Vi voglio bene, grazie.

And to Carl, thank you for everything. Lucky me.

Resources

Psychotherapy, Treatment Approaches, Support

If you've never been in psychotherapy to address childhood trauma and you're experiencing symptoms that interfere with your well-being, I suggest that you seek professional support with a trauma-informed licensed psychotherapist. As you've learned, healing from early trauma is key to healing emotional eating too.

These issues are tough to handle in isolation. People do better when they have someone to witness and support them. You can ask your medical providers for referrals or search the therapy directories below; combined, they include therapists in the United States, Canada, and internationally:

Goodtherapy.org

PsychologyToday.com

Theravive.com

Zencare.co

Licensed psychotherapists include doctorate-level clinical psychologists and master's level clinical social workers (like myself), marriage and family therapists, and mental health counselors. Psychiatrists and psychiatric nurse practitioners offer medication consultation and some also provide psychotherapy. A psychotherapist's degree is less important than their clinical experience and how you resonate with them. It's important that you find a psychotherapist experienced in working with trauma rather than a generalist. If you find a trauma-informed therapist who also is experienced with emotional eating, that's terrific. If that's not possible, however, there are other resources to address your relationship with food. For example, many therapists offer support groups for certain issues, including emotional eating. Support groups are a great way to connect with like-minded people facing similar challenges. You also can work with an intuitive eating registered dietitian or coach. Find one at: http://www.intuitiveeating.org /certified-counselors.

Dialectical behavior therapy (DBT) is a skills-based form of psychotherapy that helps people cope with overwhelming emotional states. You learn tools to develop mindful awareness, interpersonal effectiveness, acceptance of "what is," and resilience to cope. Some practitioners offer DBT groups, which are a wonderful way to learn the skills and receive additional support. (To learn how to use DBT for emotional eating, read J. Taitz's book recommended in the following pages.)

Eye movement desensitization and reprocessing (EMDR) is a psychotherapeutic treatment to help people cope with disturbing memories and the emotional distress caused by traumatic experiences. The therapist uses a technique to guide your eye movements as you hold images in your mind about the trauma you experienced. For example, the therapist may ask you to look at her finger as she moves it side to side while you think about an episode of trauma. It is believed that this bilateral stimulation helps you safely process painful trauma-based emotion. Learn more at http://www .emdr.com.

The emotional freedom technique (EFT), also called tapping, is an energy psychology technique considered a "cousin" to acupuncture. Instead of using needles, you gently tap certain energy points on your body while repeating words and phrases associated with disturbing memories or emotions. EFT is an effective self-calming tool that can help reduce emotional eating triggers, release limiting beliefs, and minimize food cravings. Learn more at http://www.emofree.com and http://www.thetappingsolution.com.

Internal family systems (IFS) is a psychotherapeutic approach that addresses the different subpersonalities or "parts" of our mind. For example, and especially with trauma, there may be a wounded part, shame-filled part, and a rageful part. IFS practitioners help the client recognize and accept their different parts, without judgment, to restore internal harmony. Learn more at https://ifs-institute.com.

Neurofeedback is a noninvasive treatment that can help improve brain functioning impacted by developmental trauma. A practitioner attaches electrodes to your scalp that are connected to a computer and monitors your brain activity. Based on the goals you have, for example to reduce anxiety, the computer provides audio-visual feedback designed to give your brain positive reinforcement to help you, over time, create new self-calming thought patterns and regulate brain wave activity. (To learn more, read S. Fisher's book recommended in the following pages.)

The polyvagal theory, developed by Stephen Porges, PhD, is a framework to teach clients about the role of the vagus nerve in the autonomic nervous system. Polyvagal theory-based strategies can help create feelings of internal safety with oneself and in connection with others. Learn more at https://www.polyvagalinstitute.org.

Donna Jackson Nakazawa offers several powerful online mindfulness and neuroscience-based writing and trauma-healing programs, including *Breaking Free from Trauma*, a 3-hour self-paced course based on a program she teaches at universities around the country, and *Your Healing Narrative: Write-to Heal with Neural Re-Narrating*™, an 8-hour self-paced course. Learn more at https://donnajacksonnakazawa.com.

PACES (Positive and Adverse Childhood Experiences) Connection is a social network that addresses the impact of trauma and other adverse experiences on individuals, families, and communities. PACES shares resources to support recovery, resilience, and inform public policy. Learn more at http://www.pacesconnection.com. (Formally named ACES Connection.)

Trauma Healing Books

Anchored: How to Befriend Your Nervous System Using Polyvagal Theory. Deborah Dana. 2021.

The Body Awareness Workbook for Trauma: Release Trauma from Your Body, Find Emotional Balance, and Connect with Your Inner Wisdom. Julie Brown Yau. 2019.

The Body Keeps the Score: Brain, Mind, and Body in the Healing of Trauma. Bessel van der Kolk. 2014.

Childhood Disrupted: How Your Biography Becomes Your Biology and How You Can Heal. Donna Jackson Nakazawa. 2015.

Complex PTSD: From Surviving to Thriving: A Guide and Map for Recovering from Childhood Trauma. Pete Walker. 2013.

The Deepest Well: Healing the Long-Term Effects of Childhood Trauma and Adversity. Nadine Burke Harris. 2018.

Getting Past Your Past: Take Control of Your Life with Self-Help Techniques from EMDR Therapy. Francine Shapiro. 2012.

Guided Imagery for Self-Healing. Martin Rossman. 2000.

In the Realm of Hungry Ghosts: Close Encounters with Addiction. Gabor Maté. 2010.

Journey Through Trauma: A Trail Guide to the 5-Phase Cycle of Healing Repeated Trauma. Gretchen Schmelzer. 2018.

Neurofeedback in the Treatment of Developmental Trauma: Calming the Fear-Driven Brain. Sebern Fisher. 2014.

No Bad Parts: Healing Trauma and Restoring Wholeness with the Internal Family Systems Model. Richard Schwartz. 2021.

Rewire Your Anxious Brain: How to Use the Neuroscience of Fear to End Anxiety, Panic, and Worry. Catherine Pittman and Elizabeth M. Karle. 2015.

Self-Compassion: The Proven Power of Being Kind to Yourself. Kristin Neff. 2011.

The Tapping Solution: A Revolutionary System for Stress-Free Living. Nick Ortner. 2013.

Therapeutic Yoga for Trauma Recovery: Applying the Principles of Polyvagal Theory for Self-Discovery, Embodied Healing, and Meaningful Change. Arielle Schwartz. 2022.

What Happened to You?: Conversations on Trauma, Resilience, and Healing. Bruce Perry and Oprah Winfrey. 2021.

What My Bones Know: A Memoir of Healing from Complex Trauma. Stephanie Foo. 2022.

Healing Your Relationship with Food Books

Body Kindness: Transform Your Health from the Inside Out—and Never Say Diet Again. Rebecca Scritchfield. 2016.

Eating Mindfully: How to End Mindless Eating and Enjoy a Balanced Relationship with Food. Susan Albers. 2012.

Eat to Love: A Mindful Guide to Transforming Your Relationship with Food, Body, and Life. Jenna Hollenstein. 2019.

The Emotional Eating Workbook: A Proven-Effective, Step-by-Step Guide to End Your Battle with Food and Satisfy Your Soul. Carolyn Coker Ross. 2016.

End Emotional Eating: Using Dialectical Behavior Therapy Skills to Cope with Difficult Emotions and Develop a Healthy Relationship to Food. Jennifer Taitz. 2012.

Health at Every Size: The Surprising Truth About Your Weight. Linda Bacon. 2010.

Intuitive Eating: A Revolutionary Anti-Diet Approach. Evelyn Tribole and Elyse Resch. 2020.

The Intuitive Eating Workbook: Ten Principles for Nourishing a Healthy Relationship with Food. Evelyn Tribole and Elyse Resch. 2017.

Lasagna for Lunch: Declaring Peace with Emotional Eating. Mary Anne Cohen. 2013.

Mindful Eating: A Guide to Rediscovering a Healthy and Joyful Relationship with Food. Jan Chozen Bays. 2017.

When Food Is Comfort: Nurture Yourself Mindfully, Rewire Your Brain, and End Emotional Eating. Julie Simon. 2018.

When Food Is Love: Exploring the Relationship Between Eating and Intimacy. Geneen Roth. 1991.

References

Hirschmann, J., and C. Munter. 1988. *Overcoming Overeating: How to Break the Diet/Binge Cycle and Live a Healthier and More Satisfying Life.* Reading, MA: Addison-Wesley.

Kingston, K. 1998. *Clear Your Clutter with Feng Shui: Free Yourself from Physical, Mental, Emotional, and Spiritual Clutter Forever.* New York: Harmony Books.

Mason, S. M., A. J. Flint, A. E. Field, S. B. Austin, and J. W. Rich-Edwards. 2013. "Abuse Victimization in Childhood or Adolescence and Risk of Food Addiction in Adult Women." *Obesity* 21, no. 12: E775–781.

Neff, K. 2011. *Self-Compassion: The Proven Power of Being Kind to Yourself.* New York: William Morrow/HarperCollins.

Orbach, S. 1982. *Fat Is a Feminist Issue II: A Program to Conquer Compulsive Eating.* New York: Berkley Books.

Roth, G. 1984. *Breaking Free from Compulsive Eating.* Indianapolis: Bobbs-Merrill.

Tolle, E. 1999. *The Power of Now: A Guide to Spiritual Enlightenment.* Novato, CA: New World Library.

Taylor, J. B. 2006. *My Stroke of Insight: A Brain Scientist's Personal Journey.* New York: Viking.

Tribole, E., and E. Resch. 2020. *Intuitive Eating: A Revolutionary Anti-Diet Approach.* New York: St. Martin's Press.

Tribole, E., and E. Resch. 2017. *The Intuitive Eating Workbook: Ten Principles for Nourishing a Healthy Relationship with Food.* Oakland, CA: New Harbinger Publications.

van der Kolk, B. 2014. *The Body Keeps the Score: Brain, Mind, and Body in the Healing of Trauma.* New York: Penguin Books.

Virtue, D. 1995. *Constant Craving: What Your Food Cravings Mean and How to Overcome Them.* Carlsbad, CA: Hay House.

Walker, P. 2013. *Complex PTSD: From Surviving to Thriving: A Guide and Map for Recovering from Childhood Trauma.* Lafayette, CA: Azure Coyote Publishing.

Watkins, J. G. 1971. "The Affect Bridge: A Hypnoanalytic Technique." *International Journal of Clinical and Experimental Hypnosis* 19: 21–27.

Diane Petrella, MSW, is a licensed independent clinical social worker specializing in childhood trauma and emotional eating. Early in her nearly forty-year career, she codeveloped the first child sexual abuse treatment program in Rhode Island. She has a private psychotherapy practice in Providence, RI. You can find out more about Diane at www.dianepetrella. com.

Foreword writer **Donna Jackson Nakazawa** is an award-winning science journalist, author of seven books—including *Girls on the Brink*—and speaker whose work explores the intersection of neuroscience, immunology, and human emotion.

Real change *is* possible

For more than forty-five years, New Harbinger has published proven-effective self-help books and pioneering workbooks to help readers of all ages and backgrounds improve mental health and well-being, and achieve lasting personal growth. In addition, our spirituality books offer profound guidance for deepening awareness and cultivating healing, self-discovery, and fulfillment.

Founded by psychologist Matthew McKay and Patrick Fanning, New Harbinger is proud to be an independent, employee-owned company. Our books reflect our core values of integrity, innovation, commitment, sustainability, compassion, and trust. Written by leaders in the field and recommended by therapists worldwide, New Harbinger books are practical, accessible, and provide real tools for real change.

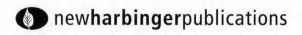 **newharbinger**publications

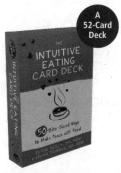
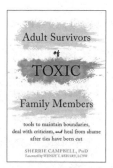
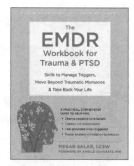
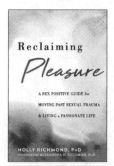
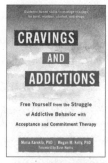
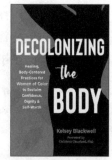

Did you know there are **free tools** you can download for this book?

Free tools are things like **worksheets, guided meditation exercises**, and **more** that will help you get the most out of your book.

You can download free tools for this book—whether you bought or borrowed it, in any format, from any source—from the New Harbinger website. All you need is a NewHarbinger.com account. Just use the URL provided in this book to view the free tools that are available for it. Then, click on the "download" button for the free tool you want, and follow the prompts that appear to log in to your NewHarbinger.com account and download the material.

You can also save the free tools for this book to your **Free Tools Library** so you can access them again anytime, just by logging in to your account! Just look for this button on the book's free tools page. ➤ **+ Save this to my free tools library**

If you need help accessing or downloading free tools, visit **newharbinger.com/faq** or contact us at **customerservice@newharbinger.com**.